HEAL
YOURSELF

BODY ~ MIND ~ SPIRIT

SANDIE GASCON

Heal Yourself
Copyright © 2021 by Sandie Gascon

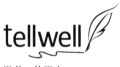

Tellwell Talent
www.tellwell.ca

ISBN
978-0-2288-5387-9 (Hardcover)
978-0-2288-5386-2 (Paperback)
978-0-2288-5388-6 (eBook)

*This book is dedicated to
my family, my greatest spiritual teachers.*

CONTENTS

INTRODUCTION

Why a Whole-Body Approach Is Needed to Heal

In modern allopathic medicine, we find doctors specializing in only one area of the body or a single aspect of health such as endocrinologists, immunologists, gynecologists, rheumatologists, and so on. Each area of the body is isolated as though they are not connected.

When I first started coaching, my business coach emphasized the importance of finding a niche. Even in the functional and holistic world there are niches. Practitioners specialize in hormones, adrenals, candida, Lyme Disease, and so forth. Just like in allopathic medicine, many holistic practitioners tend to focus on treating only one area of the body as though nothing is connected.

I thought long and hard on what my niche would be. Due to my own experience healing from chronic illness, I was unable to pick one. I knew that regardless of what symptoms or diseases are present, the entire body, mind, and spirit must be addressed as a whole because everything is connected. As you will see below, each system is important, and none can be left out.

The brain is the master organ. If it isn't balanced, nothing else will be. Sadly, the brain is left out by most practitioners. Most are not trained in balancing neurotransmitters. Few understand the genetics behind the enzymatic processes in the brain and how to analyze test results, nor have they heard of amino acid therapy to balance neurotransmitters. Amino acid therapy was my first step to healing as I was getting off of

Effexor (antidepressant); it was my catalyst. In working with hundreds of clients, I have seen balancing neurotransmitters be the missing link, which is why we will spend a lot of time discussing it.

General nutrient deficiencies need to be addressed right from the get-go as do mitochondria (our energy generation centers). If our bodies are not able to efficiently produce energy, healing will be at a standstill. Any stressors on the body deplete nutrients. Deficiencies then lead to dysfunction and imbalances, which cause the body to no longer be able to cope with stress. It becomes a vicious cycle. We interrupt the cycle by removing stress and giving the body the tools that it needs in order to repair itself. The foundation tests I use in my program will show what the body needs for both of these areas.

Detoxification pathways are the next most important part of healing. New discoveries in genetics show us how our enzymes of detoxification are impacted by our genes. Since delving into the world of genetics, my success rate and the time it takes me to help people see results have improved dramatically. Being able to customize our supplements based on our genes is an amazing scientific discovery. Milk thistle, turmeric, methyl donors, and so many other supplements are not beneficial to everyone. These popular supplements can actually do more harm than good. Many health-minded people claim they are working on their detoxification pathways, but in reality, without testing, they are throwing paint at the wall and hoping it will stick.

Many practitioners place a big emphasis on treating adrenals and sex hormones whenever a client complains of fatigue. While adrenals and sex hormones do play a role in energy levels, the saliva panel many practitioners are still using to test them is outdated. I have found that imbalances and dysfunctions in adrenals and sex hormones tend to be due to dysfunctions in other systems such as detoxification pathways, deficiencies, mitochondria, and neurotransmitters. Since adrenal function is impacted by chronic stress, fear, and depression, I prefer to first address mindset and get foundational support on board before testing adrenals and hormones. This gives the body enough time to rebalance hormones and adrenals itself with the tools we give it.

The thyroid is another area I see people concentrate on with limited success. Many doctors have not even heard of Reverse T3. In some countries, the test is not even available; as you will see in the "Thyroid" section, you cannot see a true picture of what is going on without this test. Thyroid dysfunction is a result of other dysfunctions in the body. I test it early on using a full blood panel, but as with sex hormones and adrenals, I prefer to first support other systems.

Healing the gut and detoxing from heavy metals are done last in my program because through experience, I have found gut work to be unsuccessful in most people until the rebuilding and rebalancing steps are in place. The mind needs to be in a calm state with little stress for gut work to be successful. When the stress response is chronically active, the immune response is suppressed, and it is difficult to eliminate pathogens. We need the body on board to help us remove the pathogens. Detoxification pathways must be functioning well; otherwise, killing pathogens will create a toxic burden that is too much for the body to handle, and the person will end up having to stop. The stress itself on the body would make it unsuccessful, even if they were able to complete their protocol.

Diet is another factor to increase the chances of clearing pathogens. I have found that in order for gut work to be successful, eating a ninety percent whole food diet is necessary. Many practitioners make clients go on a strict diet right away. This is rarely successful because people feel isolated and deprived. They become depressed, then at some point, they end up with feelings of shame when they binge on unhealthy foods due to intense cravings. Having time to slowly transition to a balanced diet is ideal, and my program allows for time before gut work to make this transition while we rebuild and rebalance the body.

Most people believe their gut, or pathogens like candida or Lyme, are causing their symptoms. I have found it is actually imbalances and deficiencies in the body and issues with detoxification pathways causing these issues. Once these are addressed, the symptoms go away, enabling us to easily clear up the root causes. The root causes are the overall body burden: stress, toxins, pathogens, and metals. It ends up looking like the chicken and the egg paradox: which came first? I believe stress causes dysfunction, which leads to symptoms and disease. Most practitioners try to kill the pathogens or remove the toxins by force, which often results in the person becoming sicker. Their body is unable to handle any more stress. I turn the process around and work with the body so it can heal. I remove the emotional stress, reduce toxin exposure, run tests to identify imbalances and deficiencies, aid the body in repairing detoxification, and then, when it is ready, assist in removing pathogens and metals. First, I clear parasites, protozoa, and biofilm. Then, I address bacteria in the large intestine. After that, SIBO and yeast are eliminated if still present. Last, if needed, I address any systemic pathogens. During gut work, gentle binders are used to clear metals. The body wants to be healthy; it just needs the tools and time to heal.

Here is an overview of my healing program for the average person. Some people with certain genetic mutations require another round of blood work before Phase Two to ensure detoxification pathways are functioning. They also may need further testing. These are more complex cases. I have focused on the basics of the program in this book. It is truly a whole body, mind, and spirit approach.

Phase One: Rebuild, Rebalance, and Repair
- ☐ Nutrition: slowly move to a ninety percent whole food diet
- ☐ Begin mindset training and meditation
- ☐ Order Organic Acids, genetics, and blood work testing
- ☐ Rebalance neurotransmitters
- ☐ Support mitochondria and thyroid
- ☐ Address nutrient deficiencies
- ☐ Repair detoxification pathways
- ☐ Order DUTCH Test and support adrenals and hormones
- ☐ Rerun blood work or further testing, if needed

Phase Two: Remove Stress
- ☐ Order gut tests
- ☐ Address parasites, protozoa, and biofilm
- ☐ Begin safe/gentle heavy metal detoxification

☐   Retest to ensure success and address bacterial dysbiosis

☐   Address SIBO, yeast and other systematic pathogens

How to Read This Book

This book is divided into three parts and covers my entire healing program. Part One focuses on the body and goes over testing, science, and supplements. Part Two focuses on the mind and is all about mindset training, learning to be aware of one's thoughts, and noticing how they are affecting the body. Bringing peace to the mind is vital when trying to heal from chronic illness. Here, I share tools I have discovered throughout my journey that you will need in order to shift to a peaceful, healing state. Part Two also covers how to achieve success in health, relationships, and finances. Part Three focuses on Spirit and is all about meditation and how to find your passion and purpose. Two-thirds of the book are about mindset and meditation because it is equally, if not more important to healing than the science of the body. I believe by the time you finish this book you will agree with me.

The best way to read this book is to start with "Part One: Body." Ideally, order the three foundation tests when you get to that section. While waiting for test results, work on changing your diet to a balanced, whole food diet. Instructions for this are in the "Nutrition" section. Finish reading "Part One: Body" in order to understand the full process.

Then, move to "Part Two: Mind." Once you get to the "Self-Care and Self-Management" section, take some time to apply the tips there. Then read a bit of "Part Two: Mind" each week while starting on the meditations in "Part Three: Spirit." Once you receive your test results, use the corresponding sections in the "Appendix" to assist in analysis. The test analysis sections are science-based. If you find the information is overwhelming, find a knowledgeable practitioner to help you design your protocols. Continue working on "Part Two: Mind" and "Part Three: Spirit" while implementing supplements from your test results. Then finish rereading and moving through "Part One: Body" as you complete each step.

My Journey to Health

Like most babies in the 1980s, I was not breastfed. On my baby calendar it says: "Wouldn't sleep through the night. Gave Pablum, slept better." This was at six days old. My poor gut. No wonder I would often scream for hours on end. I was fully vaccinated to the schedule at the time. Throughout childhood, my teenage years, and most of my twenties I suffered from reoccurring Strep throat infections. Antibiotics were the norm for me, usually prescribed three to four times a year.

At age seven, I had my first migraine. I still remember that day. I remember the pain. I was at my aunt's trailer. I can smell the trailer. I can see the couch and the ceiling, feel the material on my body, and hear myself screaming. My head felt like it was going to explode, and I felt so nauseous. The lights were so bright and every sound was piercing. How can a child articulate such pain that would later cripple me as an adult?

The migraines persisted and became more frequent as I got older. It took a while to realize that scents were a big trigger for me. Everyone was still smoking indoors, which did not help. I had asthma and was on multiple inhalers. When I began menstruating, I started to not sleep well; I was up most of the night and slept much of the day. I started having phases of mania that allowed me to stay up and go-go-go for days. It would be followed by a period of migraines, depression, extreme nausea, and intense cravings for junk food. I would need to be in my room with the lights out and a pillow and an ice pack on my head. The cycle would last two weeks, then repeat. I missed a lot of school. Over the years, I tried every drug on the market for migraines but had no success.

Growing up, we ate the standard American diet: meat, some veggies, and lots of pasta. I ate mostly cereal with milk. I loved candy. Those were my staples, and processed carbs were my go-to up until my mid-twenties when I discovered natural healing.

My childhood was stressful, and my teen years even more so. Stress was constant. I found solace riding my horse, C.L. Riding was my escape. I was always a bit overweight, and that contributed to insecurities and eating disorders. I started binging and purging when I was fifteen years old. I was put on Meloxicam for swelling and pain in my knees that came and went. It was worse in the cold Canadian winters.

I suffered from Raynaud's for as long as I can remember. I did not realize it was not normal until my twenties. I thought everyone's hands and feet went white when they got cold. In high school, I caught Mono and missed three months of school. I felt terrible but enjoyed not going to school. School was always easy for me, and I felt it was a waste of time sitting at a desk when I could easily teach myself from the textbook in much less time. I was blessed with an amazing photographic memory, which I had until I started drinking alcohol as a teen. I spent many weekends binge-drinking at parties.

At nineteen, I was diagnosed with Bipolar Depression. I was entering university at that time, and my goal was to be a doctor so I could find a cure for migraines. I was prescribed Effexor, as my mother was taking it and it helped her.

The Effexor stabilized the intense mood swings and reduced my migraines. I would still get them in response to scents, stress, or car rides, but the duration and intensity was reduced. The medication also turned me into a zombie. I was unable to feel many emotions, but at the time, not knowing any better, it was an improvement.

In my mid-twenties, I started thinking about becoming pregnant. I was doing research on it and came across some information on "Effexor babies." I knew how bad the withdrawals were if I missed a dose of the medication. I could not imagine a baby going through that, so I tried to get off it. Not knowing any better, I tried cold turkey. It did not work. The brain zaps and migraines were too intense. I would end up in the shower, running cold water over my body while vomiting. The doctors would not believe me when I told them what happened. "Your brain needs the medication," they said. It was then, in my third year of university, I decided I no longer wanted to be a doctor. I could not morally prescribe a drug that caused these side effects and was impossible to stop taking.

After a lot of contemplation, I decided to become a massage therapist. I had always been great at giving massages without training and figured I could be even better with training. I would still be able to help people, just in a different way. I finished my last year of university, receiving a four-year honors degree in Biomedicine, and I moved three hours from home to go to college. I was able to fast-track the three-year program to two years and skip over many courses due to my prior education. This was ideal, as I was raising and homeschooling my eight-year-old niece at the time. The reduced course load meant we could spend more time riding our horses.

In my last semester of massage therapy, right before exams, I developed a high fever and severe neck and body pain. I was brought to the hospital, where they thought it was meningitis and forced me to have a lumbar puncture. They said I could not use the phone until I did the test. It was a traumatic event. I was terrified to get the lumbar puncture and did not want to do it, but I was worried about my niece. I had left quickly, so I needed to check in with the babysitter and contact my parents so they could come help me. A stool test then revealed I had food poisoning, so the lumbar puncture had been performed unnecessarily. I was sent home and told I would get better in time. I had high amounts of Campylobacter, which caused severe diarrhea for two weeks. I lost twenty pounds. All my college testing was delayed because I was so weak. This was the turning point in my health. It had never been great before, but it took a turn for the worse.

Over the next year, I graduated from college and started work as a massage therapist. I slowly got my strength back and put the weight I had lost back on. I started to develop pain in my hands and feet. After the lumbar puncture, I started having severe pain in my back at the insertion site. I also developed numbness and weakness in both legs. The left leg was so weak and numb I could not mount a horse on the left side. I had all sorts of tests and they could not find anything wrong. I was so upset about the damage, as I had not wanted the lumbar puncture to begin with.

The following spring, I started to have a heart arrhythmia. I ended up in the hospital because my heartbeat was erratic. I was hooked up to a heart monitor. I had a missing T wave. The doctor prescribed a beta blocker. "No, thank you," I said. I already had one medication I was unable to stop taking. When I described all my symptoms, he sent me to a rheumatologist for further testing.

A few months later I saw the rheumatologist, had some tests, and was diagnosed with Lupus. As I was waiting for a diagnosis, I met someone with Lupus. At the time, I thought it was a coincidence, but now I see it as synchronicity. She was fifty years old, but she looked eighty. She told me not to take the medications. That, of course, resonated with me. She said the medications had destroyed her immune system, and her kidneys were failing. She told me to research natural remedies. The day I was diagnosed with Lupus, I said "no, thank you" to the script of Plaquenil, despite my doctor's warnings that I would die without it. I went home and started my natural healing journey.

The first thing I found was a book on healing Lupus with raw foods. I read it and believed it. I went cold turkey from a completely processed food diet to a raw food diet. As you can imagine, that did not go too well. Over the next year, I tried my best to maintain a raw food diet. I would feel so good on it but was so hungry, despite eating 4000 calories a day. I tried different fuel ratios: higher fat, higher protein, and higher carb. None of them lasted for long. I was so frustrated and angry with myself that I was unable stick to it. I kept trying, determined to find the willpower.

In June of 2012, the Effexor stopped working. It had been an extremely stressful year. Our horses had massive injuries that cost thousands of dollars, and shortly after that, my car broke down. Then the migraines returned. I was tired and unable to keep up with my already reduced workload. I had two people living in our house just to help with rent. I decided to move back with my parents.

The next year was rough. I fell into a deep depression. I tried seeing a psychiatrist. Her solution was for me to take more medications, and I didn't find she helped with talking through any emotions. Her office was also heavily scented, and I soon stopped going. Group therapy was the only other option and again, more fragrances. I went on social assistance and what little money I had went to trying raw vegan and various other diets like Paleo, AIP, low FODMAP, GAPS, and the candida diet. None were sustainable, and many made me feel much worse. Others worked only temporarily. Each failed attempt fed my feelings of depression and self-loathing.

In 2013, I came across a podcast episode by Shawn Stevenson called "4 Steps to Ensure a Disease Diagnosis Doesn't Kill You." It was about letting go of labels and changing focus to healing. There was an intense shift inside of me, as I realized I had become the disease. I would always tell people I had Lupus. It had become my identity. I was being fed by various Facebook groups, all of them focused on illness and symptoms. I had been operating in victim mentality by blaming: my parents for my poor diet, the doctors for prescribing medications, and the particular doctor for forcing the lumbar puncture. I was also blaming society and the media for promoting and allowing these foods and toxins to be made.

After the shift, I unlabeled myself from Lupus. I started stating, "My body is sending me a message. I will figure it out. I am healing. I will heal." I became determined to figure it out if it was the last thing I did. I had renewed hope and determination. I was going to reach my goal of being healthy no matter what. I began to research nonstop. I was focused on trying different diets. As mentioned earlier, some worked for a time and then I got worse, some made me super sensitive, and others just made me feel terrible.

My mom had introduced me to meditation when I first started having migraines. I had used it on and off to help with pain and staying calm, but I had strayed from it during the year of depression. With the shift in focus to healing, I got back into it. In a meditation, I asked the question: "Why am I unable to tolerate foods the same way as others do?" Eric, my boyfriend at the time (now my husband) ate whatever he wanted with no issues, and he was healthy. In the meditation, the answer came: "A healthy body can tolerate food. Work on getting your body healthy. Food is not the problem."

My research changed. I switched focus to the biochemistry of the body instead of diets. I used my training in Biomedicine, in particular my minor in Neuropsychology, to look at the chemistry of the brain. I researched the mechanism of action behind beta blockers, which I had been prescribed (and refused to take) for my heart arrhythmia.

I researched the science behind how a beta blocker works: it blocks dopamine action on the heart. The research shifted to how to naturally lower dopamine. I found out about amino acid therapy. Everything clicked. I was on an SSRI (Selective Serotonin Reuptake Inhibitor), which works by slowing the breakdown of serotonin. When serotonin goes low, dopamine goes up. I realized that all I had to do was raise my serotonin, so I started using amino acid therapy to help support my brain.

I also discovered on forums that in order to successfully get off Effexor, you needed to open the capsules and remove one bead a day. I asked my pharmacist, and he said, "No, you cannot open the capsules." He offered no other suggestions, so I opened the capsules. There were 494 beads. I remember saying to myself "This is going to take a while." I began the slow journey of going off Effexor. It took about a year and a lot of patience. It was so tempting to take out more beads. Whenever I went too quickly, I would end up having to backtrack and let the withdrawals pass, which wasted more time.

During that year, I started taking various supplements and doing cleanses to work on my liver and gut. I was researching every minute of the day, not in Facebook groups, but instead immersing myself in the science behind how the body works. Shawn Stevenson's podcasts introduced me to the world of Functional Diagnostic Nutrition (FDN). I wanted to take the course and knew that once I got better and returned to work, I would pay off my student loans and save enough money to do it. I wanted to use the tools and knowledge I was learning to help others.

I was able to get off of Effexor. It took a few months of being off it for my brain to really stabilize. I was flooded with emotions I had not felt in so long, and it took a lot of work to find balance. I was able to get the Lupus antibodies down, my energy up, and my brain healthy. I decided it was time to go back to work as a massage therapist and began the process to get my license back. I also began working locally, helping to coach people on their health issues.

The only thing I was unable to see improvement in was my skin. I had suffered from Cystic Acne since I was a teen. I tried everything and often was doing multiple things at once. It really had not bothered me when the fatigue and pain was crushing. Now that those were better, I wanted clear skin. Huge cysts on my face and back were unappealing. I decided to try lowering my estrogen, as estrogen dominance can cause skin issues. I started high doses of a supplement called DIM (Diindolylmethane), did high fat Paleo, and added in a nice, high dose ascorbic acid protocol.

It was a recipe for disaster. I ended up with pain in my urethra. I went to the doctor, who checked for infection, but nothing was there. The pain started to spread to my bladder. I did not understand, as I was doing all the right things. The pain was so bad I would have gladly traded it for what I had gone through with Lupus symptoms and migraines. A urologist diagnosed me with Interstitial Cystitis. Researching online was devastating, as I found so few people who were successful at treating it.

I was back to work. I had started my own mobile massage therapy business, and I was in high demand. I was working hard but getting through each client's appointment was torture. I often had to stop and pee once or twice a session because the pain was so intense. I often cried all through the night, sleeping with a towel between my legs because I was too tired to get up every five minutes to pee. I tried for a year to heal the IC myself, trying various herbs to sooth the bladder and following the IC diet. Nothing was helping.

Even though my student loans were still high, I decided to go further into debt and take the FDN course. I had thought about going back to school to be a naturopath, but that would take too long. I needed access to testing, and naturopaths in my province were highly regulated and couldn't order the tests I wanted. I had many theories and needed to do these tests instead of guessing.

I enrolled in the FDN course and started running tests on myself. After I finished, I continued to FDN Advanced and immersed myself in other training courses to get up to date on current testing. I learned about oxalates and sulfur. I could see my estrogen was low. I had also been ignoring my body's messages, so all along what I had been doing for my skin with diet and supplements had been hurting me. While doing high fat Paleo, I was eating so much sulfur: eggs, cruciferous veggies, nuts, seeds, and meat. I was flooding my body with sulfur and ammonia. I had also developed intense pain and gas. I thought it was my gallbladder, as I kept ending up in the hospital with either severe nonstop vomiting or diarrhea. This would cause dehydration that required IV fluids and medications to make it stop. It took me quite a while to make the sulfur and ammonia connection. Testing confirmed it was indeed the culprit, so I went to work making changes to detoxify the buildup.

While putting these last few pieces of my health puzzle together, I continued working as a massage therapist and coaching locally. I also began creating my online coaching business, Motivated 2 Heal. I had figured out the key to amazing energy, drive, and focus. Within months, I started to see a great reduction in my bladder and stomach symptoms. I listened to my body and added grains and more starchy veggies back into my diet while keeping my sulfur low. By the time I launched Motivated 2 Heal, my bladder was ninety-five percent better.

After I launched Motivated 2 Heal online, I realized I had no idea how to grow an online business. Through a Facebook ad, I found Daria Zest. I knew I needed help, so I hired her as a business coach. It was a big investment, of which I had been making quite a few already, but I knew in my gut it was the right thing to do. I initially wanted help getting my business going so I could stop massage therapy; I did not realize I was in for a complete paradigm shift.

Daria introduced me to mindset training and the Laws of Attraction. We went to work, not on my business but on my limiting beliefs. When I was not working as a massage therapist to pay the bills, or coaching clients, I was listening to different mindset books and courses. I had extra time now that I no longer had to focus on my bladder. Amazingly, after running the tests and working on the imbalances and deficiencies, my skin cleared up on its own. As I worked through my limiting beliefs, my business boomed. My whole-body approach and use of tests resonated with many people.

Just as my time with Daria was ending and we were about to leave for Florida for a month, Eric had a stroke. He was transported to St. Michael's Hospital in Toronto, where they discovered he had a subarachnoid brain bleed. He spent a week in the hospital.

It was a scary time. He was lucky to be alive. Thankfully, he was on vitamin K supplements, so he clotted quickly. The first week, I was concerned he was going to have short-term memory issues, as he would forget things he had said and done earlier. Thankfully, it only lasted a week. He could barely walk due to the blood pooling in his spine. After a couple weeks, his mobility was back to normal, but he was having intense migraines. I had started him back on supplements and introduced amino acid therapy into his regimen. When we went for his six-week checkup in Toronto, the neurologist was astonished at how quickly Eric was healing and that he had regained his function. We were able to keep the migraines at bay with amino acid therapy.

I remember when he was in ICU, I refused to leave his room. They agreed I could sleep on the floor if I stayed out of the way. One night the nurse said to me, "Go get a hotel, get some sleep. We will call you if anything changes. He is going to need you to have your energy up to take care of him when he goes home." She thought he was going to need full-time care, but I was positive he would get better. I spent most of the time there visualizing him back to health. Had it not been for my mindset training, I would have broken down.

Eric's stroke made me realize I had to start speaking up about my feelings and what was not working in our relationship. I was ready to have a baby; he was not. We had been together for a long time, and I wanted real commitment. Daria was there to help me through my limiting beliefs. I had achieved success in my health, as I was almost free of IC, except some pain during sex. My skin was clear, my online business was booming, and my clients were having great success with my whole-body approach. Now, my relationship and personal goals needed addressing.

When my time with Daria came to an end, I asked for guidance in finding my next teacher. Again, through Facebook ads, my next teacher appeared. A contest for a free ticket to Jack Canfield's *Breakthrough to Success* appeared on my Facebook newsfeed. I entered. Two days later I found out I won.

This was a big decision for me. Eric was still recovering and needed some support, and *Breakthrough to Success* was happening in Philadelphia on his birthday and our anniversary. I had also never travelled alone. I decided to face my fears and go. While there, I had huge personal breakthroughs and healed some unresolved emotional trauma that pushed my bladder to a hundred percent better. I was able to have sex again without pain. My mind was blown. I needed to incorporate mindset work and healing from emotional trauma into my program. I decided to sign up for *Train the Trainer* with Jack. It was another big investment, but my gut once again said it was the right thing to do. These tools could help me help many people.

It was worth it. I learned so much about myself going through the program, and I use the skills every day to help my clients achieve success not only in their health, but in their relationships, finances, and all other aspects of life. At the end of *Train the Trainer*, they have a Come as You'll Be Party. For this, you come as how you see yourself five years from the current time. I went to the party very pregnant, not with my first baby, but my second. The entire time, you talk and act as though you are five years into the future. It was a great experience and really put me into creation mode.

I reached a point that September that shifted my focus from achieving and building my business, to being content and present. I had done so much in a short time. Now, I wanted to sit and enjoy what I had created and focus on building a family.

Eric had undergone a vasectomy after I was diagnosed with Lupus, as I did not think I would be able to have children. We started trying to get pregnant using insemination in September 2017, and in January of 2018 after four tries, I was pregnant.

My pregnancy was tough. I started out eating well, then the nausea hit at six weeks. Luckily, I had my mindset training. I remember sitting on the couch, throwing up due to the nausea and peeing myself each time I vomited. Instead of being frustrated, I was laughing my way through it with the help of *The Big Bang Theory* episodes. I took a reduced client load during my pregnancy. My nausea lasted until sixteen weeks, but food aversions and intense cravings lasted until my baby was born.

In my last trimester, I tore my round ligament. It was more painful than giving birth. The pain lasted the entire trimester, and baby Kaiden came two weeks late. Though I was in a lot of pain, I did not suffer. Nisargadatta Maharaj says, "You do not suffer, only the person you imagine yourself to be can suffer. The observer is beyond the state of changing." Through this work, I have found that statement to be my truth. At times when the pain was immense, even if I could not find joy, I found peace and acceptance in the moment, knowing that all things will pass.

I calmly faced many fears during my labor with Kaiden. A potentially traumatizing experience ended up being the most empowering one of my life. For most of it, I labored in meditation. Kaiden was born, weighing nine pounds, ten ounces, on September 28, 2018.

I ended up losing a lot of blood during delivery. Kaiden had some trauma to his head due to me pushing for four hours. I had a long recovery, with a grade three vaginal prolapse. I was fortunate to have only one stitch from the forceps but no tearing.

There was no riding and little walking for me over the winter as I healed. It worked out well as I immersed myself in genetic courses while working with clients.

The following winter, I finished creating my mindset course despite lack of sleep. It was a big undertaking to make workbooks and record videos with a toddler. When Kaiden was about eighteen months old, his body decided to bring in a lot of teeth at once. It affected him at nighttime, which meant not a lot of sleep for me. It was during that time that the idea for this book came to me in a meditation. Each night while Kaiden was squirming and keeping me awake, more ideas flowed; the rough draft for "Part Three: Spirit" was written in two weeks. The words seemed to come from nowhere. If I did not grab them and write them down, they would disappear. I remember laughing while I was listening for ideas because whoever or whatever was sending them to me was quite unorganized. Random ideas were thrown at me that I then had to shape. I see now that the disorganization of ideas allowed the book to be created in a way that kept me from being paralyzed by fears and self-sabotage. The book started out as a thirty-day program on meditation, grew into a course on mindset, then evolved into a three-part book covering my entire program on healing the Body, Mind, Spirit.

PART ONE

BODY

Different Types of Practitioners

Most medical doctors look at the body in a piecemeal way, splitting each organ and system, then assigning it to a different specialist. Most do not look at root causes. Their goal is usually to turn off a symptom, even if the result is the body getting worse. They diagnose and treat disease, though treating disease never really means getting better. Modern medicine is sick care, not health care. There is little in the way of prevention. You can see this when you get tested for an illness and are told nothing is wrong, despite the fact that you are only two points outside of the disease range, according to their range. I just looked at my sister's blood work, and her ferritin was 8 ug/L. The normal range on her blood work was from 5–340 ug/L. She was told she was "normal," even though she was close to iron anemia and had all the symptoms. Normal is not optimal. Modern medicine does not look at optimal ranges. In Canada, the tests doctors are able to run can be affected by cuts in the medical system. Trying to get a family doctor to run a full thyroid panel is like pulling teeth. All you need is TSH (Thyroid Stimulating Hormones), according to them. If it is not normal, you can try a medication. If that fails to work, only then are you allowed to run more tests.

The medications they prescribe come with side effects. On commercials, they list side effects during scenes of people laughing and living life, with upbeat music in the background. I personally would only take a medication in life-threatening events. There is no doubt that emergency medicine is amazing and saves lives. Chronic disease management, from a modern medicine perspective, however, maintains life but at the cost of living. Sadly, there is a place for it in current times, as most people do just want to turn off the symptom and keep living life as usual. It is easier to take a pill than change one's habits and entire lifestyle. One could argue that the only reason they have those habits is because they have been conditioned by society from a young age to value them. At the end of the day, the responsibility lies with oneself.

Functional medicine doctors are medical doctors or practitioners with a Doctorate, such as chiropractors and osteopaths, that practice a more natural, holistic approach. Many still prescribe medications like antifungals and antibiotics. They believe in finding the root cause, some to the point that they will only work on the root cause and will not do any natural symptom relief. They are open to running tests. Like all practitioners, they vary in their skill and beliefs.

Health coaches, like myself, are not doctors. We do not diagnose or treat disease. We do not prescribe medications. We provide educational information and act as a guide. This book is just that: educational information that I have gathered on my journey and am sharing with you. Anything you read here is for educational purposes only. Always consult your health care provider before making changes to your diet, supplements, medications, or exercise plan.

Most health coaches have overcome some sort of health issue themselves and have years of research. It is functional medicine without the medicine. There are many different courses and trains of thought among practitioners. After healing myself, I chose being a health coach as the best fit for me. Today there are so many amazing courses out there. As a practitioner, you can pick and choose which ones jive with your approach. You do not have to get stuck in a long, expensive program that pushes one approach.

It is common for practitioners to disagree with each other, regardless of which modality they use. Each practitioner is using their knowledge and experience based on what has worked for them, and I truly believe each wants to be of service and help others heal. There are many different roads to success. Choose one that resonates with you.

The Body Bank Account

One of the most common questions I receive is, "What is the root cause of my illness?" Everyone wants to blame something: Lyme, candida, mold, root canals, antibiotics, medication, and so on. I have found the answer to be that there is never a single root cause of illness. We all start out with a reserve. I think of these reserves as our bodies' "bank accounts." Genetics and the health of our mother will determine how much of a reserve a person has in the beginning of their life. Through pregnancy and after birth, any stress we encounter makes withdrawals from the bank account. Stress includes emotional stress, physical stress, and chemical stress. Emotional stress is pretty straightforward. Physical stress will include things like injury and exercise. Chemical stress includes toxins, metals, and pathogens. Our world is a stressful place.

The majority of people eat a Standard American Diet (SAD). Kids grow up lacking nutrients. Moms are nutrient deficient, which creates more genetic mutations being expressed from the womb and beyond. If a mom's detoxification pathways, in particular methylation, are not functioning optimally, it will mean less detoxification capability for the baby. Formula fed babies start out with a propensity for leaky gut. Moms are now getting vaccinated while pregnant, and babies currently being born have the most vaccines in history.

Withdrawal after withdrawal is happening from our bodies' bank account, which quickly becomes depleted. Once the person hits zero balance and goes into debt, symptoms start occurring. The further in debt they get, the more symptoms appear, and eventually, disease is inevitable. It is no wonder we are seeing illness in increasingly younger individuals, and the rate of all diseases continues to climb. The amount of stress we face is outrageous.

By the time you start showing symptoms, the last event is what most people correlate with their symptoms and illness. In reality, it is just the straw that broke the camel's back. If it were not that case of food poisoning, for instance, then it would have been the next stressor.

That is why I don't focus on pathogens or metals in the beginning, and I do not recommend strict diets. Both of these end up stressing the body further. We need to stop making the withdrawals, or at least reduce them, and start making deposits.

Deposits are supplements, herbs, and foods that fuel us. Deposits include fueling our souls with passion, purpose, joy, and love. Stopping the withdrawals is done by removing chemicals in our environment, reducing emotional stress through mindset work, eating clean, whole foods, and in time, removing metals and pathogens. Rebuild and rebalance, repair detoxification pathways, and remove stress; these 4 Rs are critical to replenishing our bodies' bank account.

Along the process, as people go through my program and start making those deposits and start reducing withdrawals, they start to feel better. Once they get above zero balance and their symptoms go away, often people try to go back to normal lives. People start to feel good and start exercising or go back to work and quickly feel unwell again. Not only must you get out of debt, you must also take the time to build up a large reserve. Once your reserve is built up over time, only then will the body be able to handle more withdrawals (as long as deposits continue to be made on a regular basis).

Supplement Mindset

A very common complaint is, "I do not want to take pills forever; I hate taking pills." We must get one thing straight: supplements are not pills. They may come in capsules, but they are not drugs. Having a negative supplement mindset can put a damper on the healing process. Our world is pretty toxic. That is not great, empowering language, but it is reality. There are toxins in our food, toxins in our water, toxins in everything we put on our skin, and toxins in the air we breathe. We are exposed to radiation all the time. Our lives are emotionally and physically more stressful than ever before. Our food has also become depleted. Mass farming has led to foods on our supermarket shelves that no longer compare to the nutritional value in foods grown a hundred years ago.

Supplements are a blessing. We should be grateful they are readily available in multiple forms that the majority of people can tolerate. Supplements are nutrients we get from food but already broken down so our bodies can easily absorb them, even when most people suffer from poor absorption and leaky gut. Supplements come in the right form so our bodies do not have to do any conversion, which is important since many people's bodies can no longer make these conversions due to gut issues and genetic mutations that are being expressed due to stress. Herbs are a gift from the earth and not only have the ability to help us regulate different functions in the body they also help us fight pathogens and aid in healing our bodies.

When clients start to run tests, especially those who have eaten a Standard American Diet most of their lives and never supplemented, there will be a lot of imbalances and deficiencies. Without supplements, they would be up the creek without a paddle. In the beginning of working on the body, there will be a lot of supplements needed.

You will need to run tests to see what the body needs, and you will give the body those tools to do the work of healing itself. The body wants to get back to homeostasis. It really is trying to heal. The support (supplements) we put in place is meant to be kept up until the internal and external stress is removed. Once you have removed toxins, pathogens, metals, and emotional stress, you will see your need for supplements decline. Once this is done, you can reduce to a three-day per week maintenance on most supplements. Many supplements will be removed from your regimen completely, and others will be taken only as needed.

When getting started on supplements, it is of the utmost importance to begin with only one supplement at a time. When a person is very sensitive, it is best to start with a sprinkle. If you are not ultra-sensitive, it is best to start at a quarter or half of a capsule then slowly work up to the dose the body tolerates. Increase by a quarter to a half capsule per day. If ever there is a reaction, return to the last dose you tolerated without issue, then add in the next supplement. A good rule of thumb is adding in one to three new supplements per week. It is good to take a couple days off from taking supplements each week to give the body a break. Some supplements are must-haves, and those can be done daily. For me, magnesium is something I take every day.

Through this process, I place great emphasis on learning to listen to the body. It is never just about getting the supplements in; it is learning which ones the body needs and when it needs them. I am able to tell exactly what my body needs most of the time by the messages it gives me, but it has taken years of practicing and listening. This pertains to food, as well. We will go over that in more depth in the next section.

While we are talking about having gratitude for supplements, we cannot forget having gratitude for the body. So many times, people who are suffering from symptoms or illness are mad at their bodies. They are upset they cannot eat what they want or do what other people are doing. Your body is doing the absolute best it can to deal with every stressor that has been thrown at it. I cannot say that loudly enough. Your body wants to be functioning optimally. Your job is to figure out the message it is trying to send, and has been sending, for a long time. Can you imagine how frustrated it is with you because you have not figured it out? Luckily, it never actually gets frustrated with us. It just keeps on trying to heal. Show some love to your body and thank it for still being here and putting up with all the stress you put it under. Learn a lesson from it and just keep on trying.

Nutrition

As soon as I get started with a client, I have them keep a food journal so I can see how they are eating. Then I help them make a slow transition to a balanced, whole food diet while we wait for test results to come in.

There are a lot of different diets out there: vegan, raw vegan, keto, Paleo, AIP, Candida, GAPS, Low FODMAPs, SCD, just to name a few. You can spend years trying different diets. I know, because I did. I started with raw vegan and was convinced it was the right diet for me because I felt so good eating that way. It was not sustainable. I was always hungry and thinking about food. Thinking is too mild of a word. Consumed and obsessed describe it better. I could not go out to eat, so I spent most of the day doing meal preparation, trying to make some healthy dessert that would taste good and satisfy the intense hunger. I was eating thousands and thousands of calories a day. Little did I know I was doing the exact opposite of what my body wanted. Though I felt good while I stayed on the diet, when I came off, I crashed hard into full-blown uncontrollable bingeing. This was followed by feelings of immense guilt, shame, and inadequacy for not having the willpower. When I did stay on it for longer periods of time, I eventually stopped feeling good. More symptoms developed, and I started becoming more sensitive to my already limited food choices. My list of "safe" foods got smaller and smaller. The same thing happened with every diet I tried, and I tried many.

As you recall, I was hospitalized for dehydration several times. This happened when I was trying high fat Paleo. I started to develop intense stomach pain, which I thought was my gallbladder. I would be doing so great with my diet, eating all sorts of healthy fats. The pain would get intense, but I would continue following the diet. At the time, it was all the rage and deemed the healthiest way to live. Eventually, I would start to either vomit uncontrollably or have nonstop diarrhea. I remember lying in bed and being able to feel the fluid I had just drank after a liquid bowel movement move through my intestines. I would eventually end up going to the hospital to get rehydrated and medicated to stop the vomiting and diarrhea.

I would then need to eat bland for two weeks, mostly rice cakes. It was all I could keep in. Then I would add in some apple carrot juice, then chicken, carrots, and oats. Once I healed, I would go back to high fat Paleo again, because I was totally brainwashed that carbs and grains were bad for me. Just like me, many people completely ignore their bodies and follow these diets, regardless of how much worse it makes them. While writing this section, I had a client tell me she was having an Interstitial Cystitis flare. At first, we thought it was a supplement, but she had been on them for a while and was doing great. Then she said she had been trying to eat healthy after the holidays. I had her send me a seven-day food journal, and what did I see? Lots of sulfur and oxalates: eggs, almond flour, almond butter, garlic, onions, and cruciferous veggies. These are a recipe for disaster if you have IC caused by sulfur, ammonia, and oxalates. We had discussed this many times, but her previous programming kicked in, making her think she had been bad over the holidays.

It took me so long to realize that none of the diets were right. I needed to stop following diets and start listening to my body. There was and still is a war on carbs: carbs feed candida, carbs feed cancer, carbs cause this, and carbs do that. Likewise, a couple decades ago, there was a war on fat. The truth I have found is most people thrive on carbs. I have analyzed hundreds of Organic Acids Tests, and more people have trouble with fat. No wonder so many people feel so bad on low carb diets. It is because they are depriving their bodies of fuel. What people call "die off" or "toxin release" is really mitochondrial dysfunction.

It is not surprising, either. Most people grew up on the Standard American Diet. The food is easy to digest and has built-in digestive enzymes. It is high in processed carbs. When people move to a "healthy" diet, they start eating foods that their bodies have never seen and have no idea how to use. Then they completely ignore their bodies' messages, saying the food is not right for them.

"Oats are bad, grain is bad, fruit is bad, and starchy veggies are bad." I grew up eating oatmeal with toast and milk every morning for breakfast. Over the years, trying different diets, I struggled to find something to eat for breakfast. I have pictures on Facebook memories of me eating a huge plate of veggies for breakfast. I tried smoothies; eggs and bacon; and leftovers from dinner, but no matter what I did I felt terrible. But "oats are bad," so I would not allow myself to eat them. I would do these "better options" and still be tired and hungry anyway. The focus was on eating high levels of micronutrients all the time.

My body really just wanted oats for breakfast. When I listened to my body and returned to eating oats, I felt full of energy, satisfied until lunch, and had no cravings. It took a lot of mental reprogramming, as my brain was screaming: "This is bad, carbs are bad, and you are doing damage by eating oats." Talk about food phobia!

People have been eating oats and other grains without issues for thousands of years. Why is it now we are having so many autoimmune disorders, cancer, etc.? It is not the grain or the sugar; it is what we are putting into these whole foods: pesticides, GMO, preservatives, chemicals, etc. These are the causes of illness, not the food itself. Yes, certain people will have sensitivities to certain foods, and true allergies need to be avoided. However, our goal is not to live in a bubble. Our goal is to get the body healthy so it stops reacting. Whole foods are not the enemy.

Depriving yourself of your ideal fuel and limiting what you eat will only cause further stress and harm to the body. At the end of the day, we need to start listening to and respecting our bodies. We need to eat. Yes, some people thrive on fat, and some thrive on protein. The key is finding the ideal fuel ratio and avoiding your individual sensitivities, while rebuilding the body so the sensitivities go away.

Our ideal fuel ratios will change throughout the day. For breakfast, I eat oats with sourdough, spelt or millet bread that is made at a local bakery with minimal ingredients, all well sourced. I have grass - fed butter on my toast, and I also put maple syrup on my toast because it does not taste good without it. I add honey and cinnamon to my oats. Before having Kaiden, I just had oats with berries, but throughout pregnancy and breastfeeding, I needed the extra carbs for fuel. I feel fueled and full until lunch. For lunch, I often eat leftovers, a salad, or soup. Sometimes I have a treat meal for lunch.

I healed from all my health issues while having treat meals. A treat meal is anything I want to eat. It could be pizza or something from a restaurant. A treat meal is not whole foods. On my healing journey, there was no food that I gave up completely. Yes, I reduced the quantities of some, but I still had things in moderation. I realized after years on strict diets that left me feeling more sensitive, sicker, and isolated, that I was overlooking something. Why could some people eat whatever they wanted and live until one hundred years old? It did not seem to be the food or toxins. It was the fact that their bodies were able to handle the food and toxins. I needed to get my body healthy enough to handle those things. I have the desire to eat clean and fuel my body, and I want to be able to live a normal life and enjoy processed foods on occasion, without issue.

The isolation and depression from extreme diets puts a halt on healing. Life is worth living, yet I see and know so many practitioners who cannot leave their house because their diets are so strict. They then push strict diets onto their clients, creating and feeding the food phobia. They add to the guilt and shame by creating unrealistic expectations for others who are not in a position to give up their own lives and live in a bubble. These practitioners may work from home and not have to

whole food diet rarely ever lasts long term. I have developed a gradual transition that happens in three phases and has worked well for my clients:

1. In phase one, make sure your breakfast consists of whole foods. Whole foods include clean meats (from animals that are fed a species-appropriate diet without the use of drugs or antibiotics and are well cared for), veggies, fruit, whole grains, raw dairy, and minimal nuts and seeds. Breakfast really is the most important part of the day. You are breaking your fast. I teach clients to focus on foods that make them feel full and energized. Farm fresh eggs and well-sourced bacon are great for those that do well on protein. One can add some home fries if they do well with carbs. Oats with berries, cinnamon, or raw honey are great for those fueled by carbs. I love my oats and have the same thing every day. Raw milk is great in the morning to have with vitamin D3 and K2 supplements. A smoothie is a great option for those that like to skip breakfast, as is a glass of fresh juice. It seems to be easy for people to make this transition. During phase one, I have people eat what they would normally have for lunch and dinner but limit all snacks to whole food choices and stop eating after dinner if weight loss is a goal. If weight gain is a goal, then a whole food snack before bed can help put on weight. This could be protein powder, raw milk with a banana, or oats, all of which will promote rebuilding through the night. I have clients stay on phase one for as long as it takes for it to become second nature. To create a habit, it takes thirty consecutive days of doing something. During this time, I also have them start to wean off caffeine if they are drinking it. Caffeine is a drug. It is acidic and affects neurotransmitters and cortisol. From all the tests I have run over the years, when EGFR (a marker of kidney function) is low and a person gives up caffeine, it will go up on its own without any other changes. If they add caffeine back in, it starts decreasing again. Reduce multiple cups of coffee to one cup per day by cutting out a cup

13

a week. Once you are down to one cup, reduce by a quarter cup a week. Just like the transition to whole food, if done slowly, it is effective because it minimizes withdrawal.

2. In phase two, I have clients add in another whole food meal, which one is up to them. Some people like to have a whole food lunch. By dinner, their cravings might be high after a long, stressful day. Many have been using food as a reward or a way to relax. This allows them to keep this pattern while getting in a whole food breakfast, lunch, and snacks. Others prefer treat meals at lunch because they are on the go and want something fast and easy. Whatever works is the best method. This phase is maintained until it, too, becomes second nature.

3. Phase three is moving to a ninety percent whole food diet. This means doing one day of all whole foods, followed by a day that consists of one treat meal and two whole food meals. This cycle repeats, giving a person three treat meals a week. Having treat meals allows you to still have a life. I have people focus on all the good food they are eating instead of being focused on the processed foods they are having on occasion. People stick to it and heal. Yes, this goes against so many other practitioners' views, but from what I have seen, people on strict diets rarely feel better long term. Instead, they end up with more health issues, in addition to feeling isolated and miserable due to their strict diets. When you address root causes, get detoxification pathways working, and get the body strong, it should handle some treat meals without issue.

Notice I say treat meals, not cheat meals. Cheating is associated with being bad. Being human is not bad. It is good to treat ourselves. Food is such a huge part of our culture. It is everywhere and yes, we are all addicted to it. So is every animal on the planet. Most of us have eaten processed foods from a young age. Just keep it to a minimum, be gentle with yourself, and focus on the good foods you are giving your body.

I have my clients add in pancreatin at the end of all meals and ox bile at the end of high fat meals; both of these aid in digestion. When these are taken at the end of meals, the body still has a chance to make its own digestive enzymes. If it is taken at the beginning of a meal, the body will produce less enzymes. We do not want to turn off the body's production. We want to help it digest. After gut work, the enzymes are seldom needed, unless someone is eating an unusually large meal. I am not a fan of using HCL (hydrochloric acid) or betaine until it has been confirmed that H. pylori is not present. Both HCL and betaine will cause H. pylori to delve deeper into the stomach lining and become harder to eradicate. I have seen H. pylori be difficult to find with testing. Often, it fails to show up until a person has been on a biofilm buster for ninety days. Betaine also affects the methylation cycle and can be problematic for some people.

Reducing the Toxic Burden on the Body

In the "Body Bank Account" section, I discussed how stress makes withdrawals on the body's reserves. Chemical stress is a big one. Not only do we want to work on eating a ninety percent whole food diet to reduce our chemical intake from food, but we also want to reduce our exposure to environmental chemicals. This includes products we put on our skin, such as lotions, make-up, soaps, shampoos, deodorant, toothpaste, perfumes, dyes, etc. It also includes chemicals in our environment like hand soaps, detergents, dishwasher gels, and cleaning products. We are also exposed to chemicals depending on the quality of our water and air. Personally, I use a Zero filter for water; I add in trace minerals and recrystallize with a Somavedic. The Somavedic is said to reduce radiation and EMF levels in the environment. I clean my house with vinegar and essential oils. Sometimes, I use Decon 30 for mildew. All our soaps are natural. When buying natural products, check the label; you want a minimal amount of ingredients and very few words you cannot pronounce. Making sure your ducts and furnace filters are clean is important, too. We also run air purifiers with HEPA 13 filters. Exercise is also a form of stress. While healing walking and yoga are great choices.

Foundation Tests

The first three tests I start with are a genetic test, Organic Acids Test, and full blood panel. These cover neurotransmitters, detoxification pathways, nutrient deficiencies, thyroid, and mitochondria. The protocols from these tests provide the foundation of support for the body, and I put them in place before running the DUTCH Test for hormones and adrenals.

I was resistant to diving into genetics. This is because I did not like the labels people put on themselves when they saw they were more prone to disease. I also did not like the doom and gloom mentality of many of the genetics teachers. Genetics was also a challenge to understand, even with a Bachelor of Science and a long history of studying the body.

After I had Kaiden and was housebound due to prolapse, I decided to dive into genetics with a big focus on Dr. Amy Yasko's work. Genetics is now the first test I run, and if a person could only choose one test, it would definitely be genetics testing. I do not look at a lot of genes, only the ones we can impact with supplements. I like to use 23andMe because it can be read by almost every software reader available today. It is also affordable, and results are turned around quickly. The downfall is that it no longer shows MAOA (monoamine oxidase) mutations. Great Plains offers a great genetics test, but it is more expensive than 23andMe. The cost to run 23andMe plus a single MAOA test is less than the Great Plains test, so most people choose the one that is less expensive. Other common tests are tellmeGen, Heritage and Ancestry, but now there are many different companies offering genetic tests. When looking at genetics, I look at markers for neurotransmitters and detoxification, so I want to run a test that is easy to read and can be put into the different readers available such as NutraHacker, Know Your Genetics, and True Report. Most of these tests are saliva kits shipped to your home, though some may require a blood draw.

For the Organic Acids Test (OAT), I prefer Great Plains Laboratories. It has the most markers, and I personally find it easy to read. It shows bacterial and yeast markers, oxalates, mitochondrial function, neurotransmitter metabolites, and some nutrient levels. Genova offers the Organix Test, and many other companies offer their own versions. The OAT is a urine test shipped to your home and sent back to the lab. It is available to order through a practitioner, private labs, and off my website: www.motivated2heal.com.

The full blood panel shows phase three detoxification pathways, liver and kidney function, iron levels, thyroid levels, and nutrient deficiencies. I run a complete metabolic panel, complete blood count, lipid panel, iron panel and full thyroid panel, plus B12, D3, and serum homocysteine. For the blood panel, most people go to their doctors to see what they can get covered by insurance. Some doctors are more accommodating than others. There are private companies in the USA where you can order your own blood work. These vary in different areas. In countries like Canada, if your doctor refuses to order it, you will need to see a naturopath.

Now is the time to order these tests. Once you have results in hand, use the corresponding sections in the "Appendix" to assist you in your self-analysis. Mitochondria support is also covered in the "Appendix." While you wait for your test results, you can continue reading "Part One: Body" to get a full sense of the program or head over to "Part Two: Mind" to begin mindset training.

Balancing Neurotransmitters

The most important place to start is, of course, the brain. Our brain is the master control. If it is out of balance, everything is out of balance. Society has us all in go-go-go mode, chasing success and running on the hamster wheel. We must have a good career, raise kids, have hobbies, have good relationships, and remember to exercise. It is non-stop. It is no wonder our brains need more support than ever before. Most people are prone to quickly burning through serotonin. I do not think it is a coincidence that the majority of our population is on an antidepressant. Chronic pain? Here is an antidepressant for that. Abnormal periods? Here is an antidepressant for that. If you have a symptom the doctors are unable to explain, you can be sure they

Big Pharm!

will prescribe an antidepressant for it. Selective Serotonin Reuptake Inhibitors are the most commonly prescribed antidepressants. SSRI is a fancy name for "slows the breakdown of serotonin." If we know most people burn through serotonin quickly, then why not just give the body the tools it needs to make more serotonin? The pharmaceutical industry cannot patent that. Instead, they have developed drugs that change the receptors in the brain, are hard on the liver, and leave lasting effects on some people when they try to stop taking them.

Anxiety is a huge factor when it comes to health issues. Doctors may say it is all in your head and prescribe an antidepressant for depression or a benzodiazepine for anxiety. If you are on medications, it is best to work with a practitioner. Never stop your medications cold turkey. "Part Two: Mind" will include a full explanation of the impact our thoughts have on our bodies. Mindset work and supporting our brain are key parts of the healing journey.

For most people, increasing their serotonin levels has the biggest benefit on their health. Serotonin brings peace, balance, and relaxation. Getting serotonin elevated puts the body into a healing state.

I have found that many people are addicted to the high dopamine state. High dopamine brings drive, motivation, and focus. It feels good, but the body cannot stay in that state forever. When the person crashes and can no longer stay in the rat race, they seek a return to that high level of dopamine through drugs, over-exercising, over-working, sex, and other fixes. The problem is, that when the body is depleted, we need that energy to heal. Energy must be conserved. Resting and healing is where focus should be, which is why I do not recommend boosting dopamine too much until the body is ready. Remember the body bank account. We want to build up our reserves before boosting dopamine.

Amino acid therapy uses precursors to neurotransmitters to rebuild levels and balance the brain. Precursors are the building blocks to making neurotransmitters. Cofactors are the nutrients needed for our enzymes to function and produce the neurotransmitters from the precursors. First, we want to get our cofactors up. The three important key players are magnesium, P5P (pyridoxal-5-phosphate), and zinc.

1. Magnesium: For magnesium, bisglycinate is the most absorbable form. Some people do not tolerate glycine. If that is the case, try malate or threonate. Citrate is not well-absorbed, and taurate can be an issue for those with active CBS mutations. (See "Genetics" section in the "Appendix" for more information on this mutation.)

2. P5P: P5P is active vitamin B6. It can cause detoxification issues, and some people may be sensitive to it. A sprinkle is all that is needed for sensitive individuals. A good dose to work up to is 25 mg.

3. Zinc: I have found zinc orotate to be the most absorbable form. Picolinate is good if you cannot get orotate, which can be difficult to find in some countries. Start with a low dose, as zinc can cause detoxification reactions. I will never forget the first time I took zinc. I took 100 mg. Within thirty minutes, I got very nauseous, then I started throwing up. It was not long before I had explosive diarrhea and the worst migraine ever. I felt like I was going to pass out. I had to lie in bed for hours until it passed.

The precursor to serotonin is 5-HTP (5-Hydroxytryptophan) or tryptophan. The Organic Acids Test will tell you if your quinolinic acid is high. If it is, you are not efficiently converting tryptophan to serotonin. Quinolinic acid is a neurotoxin and causes brain fog, migraines, depression, and fatigue. If your quinolinic acid is high, you will want to avoid tryptophan and use 5-HTP to bypass that step. High quinolinic acid indicates pathogens and a lack of cofactors. 5-HTP is my supplement of choice. The dose I have found works best for most people is 100-200 mg, one to three times per day (though some people need more and some need much less). The MAOA (monoamine oxidase) enzyme is responsible for the speed at which we break down serotonin. People who are MAOA -/- will need more serotonin support, +/- less and +/+ should need very little. I have seen many people who are MAOA +/+ need a lot because their mutation is not active. See the "Genetics" section in the "Appendix" for more in-depth information on gene status and interpretation.

Always start on a low dose of supplements and work your way up. You can also use St. John's Wort to slow the breakdown of serotonin so that less 5-HTP is needed. It acts as a natural SSRI. Not everyone does well on the herb, though. I tend to use herbs less often because they do act more like a drug, just a nontoxic one. Most people do well taking 5-HTP each day for maintenance and increasing it during times of stress. For some people, 5-HTP makes them sleepy, and for others, it gives them energy. I have clients start out by taking it at 4:00 p.m. That way if it makes them tired, bedtime is not far away. If it gives them energy, they have some time to burn it off before bed. Then they can adjust the dose and time based on how they feel. I personally cannot take it past 5:00 p.m. If I do, I will be up most of the night.

When I first got off Effexor, I was taking 5-HTP daily. As I started to do mindset work, I needed it less and less as I was no longer reacting to stressful events in my life. Since having Kaiden, I have found I need it more often due to lack of sleep. It keeps my brain supported. The COMT (Catechol-O-methyltransferase) enzyme is responsible for the speed at which we break down dopamine. I am COMT +/+ which means I break down dopamine very slowly and am prone to high dopamine levels. This would cause mania in the past because my serotonin was very low with my MAOA -/- status. The high dopamine would last a couple weeks, then I would completely crash into depression and have migraines as I burned through the dopamine. As my dopamine rebounded, I would cycle back to mania. By understanding my genetics and that methyl donors push my dopamine higher, I now know that I must keep my serotonin up to balance the dopamine and keep my methyl donors low to prevent dopamine dominance. Methyl donors are molecules that contain and donate a methyl group. Common ones are methyl B12, methylfolate, betaine, and methionine.

As a note, 5-HTP is listed as "do not take while pregnant or breastfeeding." I have taken it throughout both. There really are no studies on most herbs and supplements during pregnancy, which is why the warning is on the labels. Somehow it is okay for a pregnant or breastfeeding mother to inject toxins into her body, take medications that are hard on the liver and change the brain; however, a supplement derived from what the body already naturally produces or gets from food is terrible. It does not make sense to me. I choose to support my body. At the end of the day, it is your body and your choice. Personally, I would prefer to take a supplement than medication.

For people who are COMT -/-, increasing dopamine is usually required to prevent depression and to increase focus. They burn through dopamine quickly. If metabolites are low on an Organic Acids Test, it indicates not enough cofactors and precursors. Using DLPA (D-L phenylalanine), tyrosine, or macuna will help boost dopamine, and ginkgo biloba will slow breakdown. I like to start with DLPA, as it can also boost endorphins. Work up to 2 grams in the morning and/or early afternoon. If there is no effect, switch to tyrosine. If there is still no effect, add in macuna.

Finding passion and purpose and setting goals is the most effective way to boost dopamine. To achieve the best results, support the brain and work on passion and purpose.

If a person is suffering from anxiety, I do not boost dopamine until mindset has been addressed and anxiety support is on board; otherwise, dopamine will convert into adrenaline and fuel the anxiety fire. The more we use one pathway or thought pattern, the more ingrained it becomes. Where attention goes, connections grow in the brain. Learning to change thought patterns takes time and commitment.

For anxiety, balancing gamma-aminobutyric acid (GABA) is important. Symptoms people associate with anxiety include heart palpitations, shortness of breath, flushing, and shaking. Mutations on the GAD (glutamate decarboxylase) enzyme will cause less conversion of glutamine to GABA. Glutamic acid is very excitatory. People who have this mutation will not tolerate sources of glutamate in their diet. GABA does not cross the blood-brain barrier. Leaky brain has been theorized, as many people report that supplementing GABA does help them. If plain GABA does not work, using liposomal GABA may help. This is a good option for people who do not have issues with sulfur, as liposomes are sulfur based. Herbs like passionflower, hops, and valerian all increase GABA.

It is good to keep GABA or GABA-boosting herbs with you if you are prone to panic attacks. The act of recognizing the anxiety and taking a supplement is a good step in interrupting the thought pattern responsible for the anxiety.

Oxalates

The amount of oxalates we are consuming is important to our health. Oxalates or oxalic acids are found in humans, plants, and other animals. Oxalates are very acidic and have sharp edges when they form into crystals. When they get into the joints, bladder, kidneys, and eyes, they do damage. Symptoms of oxalates are joint pain, burning when urinating, painful bowel movements, crystals, kidney stones, IC, and fatigue. They can interfere with your brain's ability to produce neurotransmitters and contribute to brain fog, depression, and anxiety. They can cause frequent urination and fibromyalgia.

Oxalates prevent mineral absorption and end up causing deficiencies. Oxalates also impair mitochondrial function and bind to heavy metals and prevent their detoxification. Oxalates decrease glutathione levels and cause neurotransmitter dysfunction. They can also cause imbalances with biotin, copper, and sulfate.

Usually oxalates are bound to calcium, but they can bind to anything like magnesium, copper, and heavy metals. When unbound in the body, due to an excess being absorbed or created, they wreak havoc. When they bind in the gut to minerals, they prevent them from being absorbed. We get oxalates from plants we eat, and our bodies can make their own oxalates. In plants, they are a defense mechanism, as they are poisonous if eaten in high amounts. If you have yeast overgrowth or other infections, they will contribute to a higher oxalate load because yeast, bacteria and even protozoa can produce oxalates.

When oxalic acid levels are high in foods, the oxalates will prevent minerals from being absorbed. For example, spinach is extremely high

Spinach?

in oxalates. It is thought to be a super food because of its high nutrient density. This may be the case, but those nutrients are not absorbable because of the oxalates. Instead, the excess oxalates that do not bind to minerals and get excreted are deposited into joints, tissue, etc., and cause damage. Many people switch to a "healthy" plant-based diet that is high in oxalates and end up developing even more health issues.

How you process and detoxify oxalates depends on your health and your genetics. Some people can tolerate them fine. I believe, in general, if you consume too many oxalates, you will run into problems over time, especially if combined with other factors discussed below.

We process oxalates in three ways. The first way is we excrete them before they are absorbed. For example, we eat high oxalate foods with insoluble calcium, and the oxalates are bound in the gut and passed in our stool instead of absorbed. The second way we process oxalates is through our kidneys. Oxalates that find their way into our bodies will pass through the kidneys when the body has enough tools to detoxify them. The third way we process oxalates is we develop a bacterium in our gut that can break down oxalates, so they are not absorbed. Sadly, the overuse of antibiotics can reduce or wipe out these bacteria known as Oxalobacter formigenes.

We get a buildup of oxalates when: we consume too many oxalates without any insoluble calcium to bind to them; the body starts to produce too many of its own; we develop deficiencies in certain nutrients that are needed to detoxify oxalates; Oxalobacter formigenes become depleted; and pathogens produce too many oxalates.

If you have oxalate overload, you do not want to quickly cut out all oxalates from your diet, as it can cause "oxalate dumping." This is when the body attempts to release its accumulation of oxalates; it is painful and can cause damage to tissues. We want to slowly move from consuming foods in the "super high" oxalates to the "very high" oxalates categories below. You want to reduce your oxalate load by only five to ten percent every month. This is safe and prevents dumping. A good first step is to add in supplement support without changing the diet too much.

There are many different charts for oxalates. The chart I use is from my own experience with detoxifying oxalates that caused my IC. Soaking and boiling foods helps lower the oxalate content but is not enough to lower the super high category. The super high foods should be avoided by everyone. They are fine occasionally, as a treat a few times a month, if a person is not having symptoms of high oxalates. In healing myself and my clients I have found that when raw milk and nutrient support are added in, a person does not have to go to a low oxalate diet. Completely avoiding "super high" oxalate foods and having raw milk with "very high" oxalates, plus allowing the body time, is enough to heal. I have found going to a low oxalate diet to be too restrictive.

Super High Oxalates Category

☑ Spinach   ☐ Swiss Chard   ☐ Soy

☐ Rhubarb   ☑ Almonds   ☑ Plantains

☐ Buckwheat   ☐ Amaranth   ☑ Sesame Seeds

☑ Cashews   ☑ Peanuts   ☑ Dark Chocolate

☑ Carob   ☐ Beet and Beet Greens

Very High Oxalates Category

☑ Eggplant ☐ Artichokes ☑ Okra

☑ Potatoes ☑ Sweet Potatoes ☑ Blackberries

☑ Citrus ☐ Figs ☑ Kiwi

☐ Pomegranate ☑ Beans: ☑ Nuts and Seeds:
　　　　　　　　　Anasazi, Navy,　　Pecans, Brazil Nuts,
　　　　　　　　　Pink, Pinto,　　　Hazelnuts, Pistachios,
　　　　　　　　　Red, White　　　　Macadamia Nuts, Pine
　　　　　　　　　Adzuki, Black,　　Nuts, Walnuts, Hemp,
　　　　　　　　　Cannellini　　　　Chia

Herbs and Spices high in oxalates that should be used in moderation:

☐ Allspice ☐ Caraway Seeds ☐ Cinnamon

☐ Clove ☐ Cocoa Powder ☐ Cumin

☐ Curry Powder ☐ Ginger ☐ Onion Powder

☐ Turmeric ☑ Black/Green Tea

High Sulfur Foods: Use caution as consuming too many high sulfur foods will cause oxalate dumping. High sulfur should be avoided with Interstitial Cystitis. One to three total servings per week of these foods is safe.

- ☐ Eggs
- ☐ Nuts and Seeds
- ☐ Broccoli
- ☐ Cauliflower
- ☐ Asparagus
- ☐ Onion
- ☐ Garlic
- ☐ Cabbage

Most people eat around 100 mg of oxalates per day. When going plant-based, this number can go into the thousands. The average lethal dose is 10-15 grams. I always think of oxalates when people are eating high levels of plant foods and not feeling better. I use the Organic Acids Test to confirm oxalates as an issue. The only issue with testing is that sometimes we get a false negative because the person does not have the ability to detoxify the oxalates.

The following supporting nutrients are essential to detoxifying oxalates:

- ☐ Vitamin B6 is important to detoxify oxalates but adding in vitamin B6 is not a good idea as many people cannot convert it to P5P. P5P is the preferred form. If a person has IC, adding in P5P can irritate the bladder. Start at a sprinkle of P5P, and if that is all you can tolerate, that is fine. Take P5P with food. More is not better when it comes to supplementing. Listening to the body trumps all.
- ☐ Vitamin B1 helps to detoxify oxalates. Benfotiamine is the active, fat-soluble form of B1 and is absorbed best.
- ☐ Vitamin C, aka ascorbic acid, can convert to oxalates. This was a big contributor to me developing IC. At the time, I was using high dose ascorbic acid therapy to clear my skin. Vitamin C in the presence of high copper will convert to oxalates. I had a copper IUD for five years. I do not use more than 250 mg of ascorbic acid at a time. It is best to use whole food vitamin C if you think you have an issue with oxalates or copper.

- ☐ Ornithine helps with detoxification of oxalates by supporting the urea cycle.
- ☐ Glucosamine sulfate can be used to compete with the binding sites if you have no issues with sulfur and are going slowly to prevent dumping.
- ☐ If you have vulvodynia, use emu oil to help soothe the vagina.
- ☐ Chanca piedra can be used to break up oxalate stones.

To get rid of oxalates, we reduce consumption, prevent absorption, reduce internal production, and aid detoxification. Slowly move to a lower oxalate diet by reducing oxalates by five to ten percent per month to avoid excessive pain from dumping. Use calcium to prevent absorption. Oxalates compete with other minerals, so take other mineral supplements at a meal other than your higher oxalate meals. If you are going to have some chocolate, have it with raw milk or plain calcium citrate. I prefer raw milk over calcium citrate, as it is full of nutrients and a great source of energy. Citrate has been thought to cause further copper imbalance, as it can lower ceruloplasmin (our major copper-transporting protein), so I like to keep it in moderation. It is a good idea to run a copper zinc test from Great Plains to check your levels.

Thyroid

When you get a thyroid panel, you will be told you are either hypothyroid, hyperthyroid, or normal. Remember, normal does not equate to optimal; we are looking for healing opportunities. Always compare your numbers to the optimal ranges in the "Blood Analysis" section in the "Appendix."

Hyper is too much thyroid hormone. Symptoms of hyperthyroid are irritability, anxiety, racing heart, diarrhea, hair loss, weight loss, hyperactivity, and irregular heart rate. Hypo is not enough thyroid hormone. Common symptoms are fatigue, depression, hair loss, feeling cold, weakness, weight gain, and trouble losing weight. It is impossible to diagnose yourself by symptoms, as many symptoms overlap. Often, you can have these symptoms and it is not even the thyroid itself. I had many of these symptoms, and my thyroid was functioning optimally. Always get tested.

I often hear from people that their doctor said their thyroid was fine. If you go to a modern medical doctor, they will most likely test only your TSH levels. If you are in the normal range, which is 0.45–4.5 mU/L (some ranges are even higher), you will be considered fine. The ideal TSH range for most people is between 0.5–2.0 mU/L. If higher and not addressed, it will not be long until you get to the disease state. Best to address it now and get into optimal ranges.

If you are outside of the normal range, doctors will most likely prescribe levothyroxine for hypothyroid. This is artificial T4. It will bring the TSH level down nicely. Most people do not convert the artificial drug into free T3. You can have a good TSH because of the medication and still have low free T3 levels because of the lack of conversion. The medication is just tricking your brain. Since doctors do not usually test anything other than TSH, they do not see the lack of conversion. Your free T3 levels are the best indicator of hyperthyroid versus hypothyroid. Make sure to get a full thyroid panel.

The next important thing to look at is reverse T3 (rT3). Most doctors do not even know what it is or that they can order it. In some countries, the test does not even exist. In Canada, these tests are sent to the USA. If your reverse T3 is above 15 ng/dL, it means your body is inactivating your thyroid hormone. If you take NDT (Natural Desiccated Thyroid) with a high reverse T3, you will end up driving rT3 up further.

Thyroid antibodies are very important. The TPO and TBG are the Hashimoto's antibodies. The normal ranges are higher than optimal ranges, so if you run the full thyroid panel as a preventative measure, you can often see an issue starting and prevent it from turning into a disease. The TRS and TRAB antibody tests most likely will not be performed unless you have clinical signs of hyperthyroidism.

If you are producing too much thyroid hormone, you do want to see your practitioner and understand what to look for in a thyroid storm. It is rare, but it is life-threatening. Symptoms are high fever, high blood pressure, high heart rate, and seizures. Work with a practitioner if you are hyperthyroid. Reducing stress is one of the best things you can do for hyperthyroidism, as cortisol dysfunction and hyperthyroidism go hand in hand. External and internal stress need to be eliminated. Lifestyle changes, addressing emotional issues, reducing toxins, reducing pathogens, and supporting detoxification pathways all help with hyperthyroidism. Carnitine, lemon balm, and immune modulators like Moducare can help with hyperthyroidism also.

For hypothyroidism, you must also address your sex hormones, adrenals, mitochondria, neurotransmitters, and detoxification pathways along with addressing your thyroid. Often, addressing these other issues will be enough to kick the thyroid back into gear. I like to run the full blood panel (that includes the thyroid) right away in my foundation tests but only add in cofactors to help the thyroid for the first few months. After the foundation protocols are on board, I run a DUTCH Test and address sex hormones and adrenals. When that protocol is on board, I rerun the thyroid panel to see if there are improvements. There usually are. If there are no improvements and the person is still experiencing fatigue, then I think about adding in NDT if reverse T3 is below 15 ng/dL. Once you start thyroid hormones, it can be difficult to get off them. You are telling the brain there is enough, so it stops stimulating the thyroid, and the thyroid stops producing hormones. When you try to go off the hormones, the thyroid often fails to kick back in even though it has the tools to do so.

The other thing that often happens when people assume the thyroid is the cause of their fatigue and go straight to treating it is that they cannot tolerate the NDT. If you have not worked on adrenals, sex hormones, liver, neurotransmitters, and mitochondria, you may find you get more symptoms of fatigue or feel like you are hyperthyroid, even if blood work isn't showing it.

Before going on NDT, it is important to support the thyroid with cofactors and precursors. These include selenium, molybdenum, iodine, and other minerals, along with tyrosine or DLPA for those with no COMT mutation or just one mutation. Try this for at least three months while supporting the other systems before trying NDT. You may find you do not need it. Your thyroid will often balance itself. If thyroid antibodies are high, start on immune modulators. You may want to get on NDT right away in that case, as NDT can often stop the immune response.

If you are on Levothyroxine, do not try to stop your medication cold turkey. You want to work with a practitioner to switch over to NDT. There are many different options via prescriptions. The current consensus from the website, Stop the Thyroid Madness (a leader in thyroid resources) at the time of writing this book is that Armour thyroid is working the best. There are also over the counter forms of NDT available. Thyrovanz and Thyrogold have the best reviews. Often formulas change, and medications become less effective. Always visit the Stop the Thyroid Madness website to keep up with the best current options.

If your reverse T3 is high, NDT most likely will not help you, as any NDT will be inactivated and will be converted into rT3. If this is the case, you will want to work on balancing the other systems. Doing so will help with symptoms. Then move to parasites and protozoa, as they are often a trigger for the autoimmune issues. The rT3 should come down after the internal and external stress are removed. If it is not decreasing and you want relief, you can do a T3 flush. You will need to be working with a practitioner for this, as thyroid levels need to be monitored, and only a medical doctor can prescribe T3. The thyroid does not function as an individual organ. The body functions as a whole, so work on everything together.

Detoxification Pathways

Our liver is an amazing organ. Some liver functions include: storing sugar, regulating blood sugar, producing and storing protein, producing bile to aid in fat digestion, regulating and metabolizing hormones, neutralizing free radicals, storing vitamins, minerals, and other nutrients, and recycling and producing red blood cells. Our focus will be on its ability to detoxify toxins, chemicals, hormones, and neurotransmitters. Important tests to run include homocysteine, B12, folate, genetic testing, Organic Acids Test, and full blood panel. See the corresponding sections in the "Appendix" for assistance in analyzing your test results.

Signs of liver dysfunction include hormonal imbalance, abnormal fat metabolism, obesity, histamine issues, slow metabolism, acne, rashes, acid reflux, nausea, indigestion, IBS, depression, brain fog, headaches, migraines, immune dysfunction, allergies, chemical sensitivities, food sensitivities, chronic fatigue syndrome, fibromyalgia, recurrent infections, blood sugar problems, and so many others. Detoxification pathways play a role in all symptoms. Since so many symptoms overlap, it is best to test and see what the body needs. There is usually never one cause of illness, but rather, many. A whole-body approach is needed.

Though we say "liver" for detoxification, detoxification does happen in other cells in the body but is highly concentrated in the liver. There are three phases of detoxification. Phase one gets detoxification rolling using CYP (cytochrome p450 enzymes). From here, toxins go to phase two for extra processing. Phase two has seven subphases: sulfation, glucuronidation, glutathione conjugation, acetylation, amino acid conjugation, methylation, and sulfoxidation. Phase three is the removal of toxins from the body through the kidneys, skin, and bile (which leaves through the bowels). For an in-depth look at the science of the detoxification pathways, see the "Detoxification Pathways" section in the "Appendix."

The DUTCH Test – Adrenals and Sex Hormones

I like to get the protocols from the Organic Acids Test, genetics, and blood work, plus mindset training and a balanced whole food diet on board before running a DUTCH Test. It usually takes two to four months to get that foundation in place. This gives the body a chance to regulate adrenal and sex hormone levels with all the support on board for the other systems. Many times, a person comes to me with a DUTCH Test. When I compare DUTCH Tests before and after the foundation protocols and mindset work is in place, there is always a huge improvement in the second test as the body utilizes the new resources to create balance. Usually, little support is needed when done in this order. We still check though, to ensure the body has all systems supported before gut work. The DUTCH Test can be broken into three parts: the adrenal portion, the hormone portion, and the other markers portion.

The other markers include melatonin and some markers shown on the Organic Acids Test: two B6 markers, one glutathione marker, a B12 marker, a dopamine metabolite and norepinephrine metabolite marker, and a marker for oxidative stress. This is good to see if any other support is needed or if support needs to be changed from the Organic Acids Test.

If you have your foundation in place, it is time to order your DUTCH Test. For this test, urine is collected four to five times per day. It is best to read the instructions when the kit is received, as there are foods to avoid. How you use the test will depend on whether you are looking at baseline levels or wanting to see how a hormone or supplement is affecting the body. For baseline levels, it is best to stop supplements for three to five days prior to testing. For specific instructions on testing bioidentical hormones, refer to the DUTCH Test educational videos at dutchtest.com. This test is quite complex when it comes to all the patterns that can present. I will cover some basic patterns and baseline testing in the section on "DUTCH Test Analysis" in the "Appendix."

Heavy Metal Detoxification

I personally don't use heavy metal testing early in my program, as I have found that often we cannot see a true picture of body burden until we begin to detoxify. I also do not use chelators like DMSA or EDTA, as I have seen damage caused by them and believe detoxification should be done at the body's pace. I also like to have detoxification pathways and the body supported before adding in any binders for metals. Instead, I add them in during gut work, which is toward the end of my program. If people want, they can test metals through hair, urine, and/or stool to monitor how detoxification support changes their levels. The clients

I have worked with almost always see results before doing any heavy metal work, so spending the money on gut testing is usually what they choose. Personally, on my healing journey, I did not do any heavy metal detoxification. I decided because I felt so amazing, it was time to get pregnant, so I stopped all detoxification months before trying to conceive. I focused only on supporting my body, repairing detoxification, and gut work and I was able to reach a level of health I never thought possible. Once I am finished breastfeeding, I will most likely do some gentle binders like Zeobind, Cytodetox, TRS, and Biosil, to work on metals. Those are the binders I add in during gut work with clients.

The Gut

Before moving to gut work, it is imperative to have these steps in place to increase the chance of success. You need to have detoxification pathways supported, have decreased emotional stress through mindset work, follow a balanced whole food diet and have support in place for imbalances and deficiencies.

Once the rebuilding and repair phase is complete, gut testing comes next. The first focus is on parasites and protozoa. It is very common for me to hear, "I ran a stool sample, and it did not show any parasites or protozoa." Most stool samples give false negatives. This is due to the lack of sensitivity of the test and the life cycle of these pathogens. They often are not shedding at the time of testing. To increase chances of seeing them in a stool sample, I use a biofilm buster. My favorite is Fibrenza. Slowly work up to two to three capsules upon rising and before bed on an empty stomach. Once the full dose is achieved, count two weeks and then test.

My favorite tests are Parawellness and GI Map. I have had the best success detecting parasites and protozoa with them. The Parawellness is a standard stool sample via microscopy and culture. It is a smaller lab, and I find they give attention to detail. The GI Map from DSL is a leader in PCR (genetic) testing. It tests for many parasites and protozoa, and it also looks for H. pylori, opportunistic bacteria, viruses, immune triggers, normal flora balance, secretory IgA (a measure of immune response in the gut), anti-gliadin (immune response to gluten), glucuronidase (high levels show issues with estrogen and a need for calcium D glucarate), and other things.

I ideally run both Parawellness and GI Map, but if finances are an issue, I would just run Parawellness to start, as it has shown in my experience to be the best for picking up the parasites and protozoa. I like to address these first because they really are not meant to be in our GI tract, and many other pathogens can live in their biofilm. Biofilm is a substance that surrounds pathogens, making them more resistant to being killed. It is important to address biofilm in pathogen protocols. If one fails to do this, they are just killing the free load of pathogens, and as a result, the pathogens in the biofilm survive and become resistant. I maintain the same dose of Fibrenza during my pathogen protocols.

Another reason why tests give false negatives is incorrect test preparation. For two weeks prior to testing, there should not be any ingestion of antimicrobials, immune boosters, probiotics, or binders. There should also be no enemas or flushes.

In all the hundreds of tests I have performed, I have had only three people's results come back negative for parasites and protozoa on both GI Map and Parawellness. For one of those individuals, these issues were detected in the next round of testing after the person had been on a biofilm buster for two months during their protocol. The other two had done very in-depth parasite protocols prior to starting with me.

After testing, stop taking the biofilm buster until the results come back. Taking a biofilm buster without antimicrobials puts a lot of strain on the body, as it must work to keep all the newly liberated pathogens in check. Once test results are in and a protocol is underway, then biofilm busters are resumed.

If you have completed the rebuilding and rebalancing phase, you can order a Parawellness test kit from their website. A GI Map must be ordered through a practitioner.

During gut work, your supplement support from the rebuilding, rebalancing, and repair phase is maintained. Liver flushes are done monthly, and coffee enemas are done once or twice a week to support phase three detoxification by removing toxins in bile. Saunas and castor oil packs can be added in one to two times a week to aid in detoxification, if needed. You can find instructions on how to do a liver flush in the book, *The Amazing Liver and Gallbladder Flush* by Andreas Moritz, and coffee enema instructions are available online.

H. pylori, if present, it is best to address it first. It can be addressed on its own for a sensitive person or in combination with the protozoa protocol, as long as the detoxification reactions are tolerable. Mastic gum, L. reuteri probiotic, matula tea and a product called PeptiMycin from Holistic Heal are my favorite. The dose and length of time taken will depend on how high the H. pylori levels are on the GI Map and how many virulent factors are present. The higher the levels, the longer and stronger the protocols. The entire household should be addressed, as H. pylori is contagious. It is also important to change toothbrushes.

For parasites and protozoa protocols, I like to use one to two antimicrobials and change them every month for a total of three months. After that, retesting occurs fourteen days after finishing the protocol. If successful, a two-month break is given to the gut before moving on to bacteria balancing. Follow the above test preparation for retesting.

Common herbs I like to use for parasites and protozoa are artemisia, clove, black walnut, and black seed oil. Products I like are Raintree AP, Designs for Health Microbe X, Bioray Artemisia and Clove, Ayush AP Mag, Mimosa, Paracid Forte, Microbe Formulas, Natromycin, Paradex, Paragard, Intesticlear, and Humaworm. I like to use SIBO-safe spore-based probiotics along with S. boulardi and rotate those daily. See the "SIBO" section for more details. I also add in zeolites like Toxaprevent or Zeobind to mop up toxins in the gut and aid in moving metals.

If the protocol is not successful, a two-month break is given before doing another three-month protozoa protocol with different antimicrobials. Currently, about eighty percent of my clients clear up on the first protocol, fourteen percent of people on the second, and I have only had a few clients need a third round.

Once protozoa are cleared, bacteria balancing is next. I like to use Biocidin, Oliverex, and olive leaf as broad spectrum antibacterials; neem for prevotella; and goldenseal and Manuka honey for staphylococcus overgrowth. The goal is to get numbers low on retesting and have GI symptoms significantly decrease after gut protocols. If symptoms are still present, move on to SIBO.

SIBO

SIBO stands for Small Intestinal Bacterial Overgrowth. It happens when good bacteria from the large intestine overgrow in the small intestine. These bacteria start to break down plant matter too early, releasing large amounts of gases that traverse the long, small intestine. These gases cause pain, bloating, cramps, diarrhea, and constipation. The bacteria consume our nutrients and also decrease fat and carb absorption. They excrete acids, damage villi, and loosen tight junctions, which cause intestinal permeability (leaky gut).

There are three types of SIBO: hydrogen, methane, and hydrogen sulfide. Diarrhea is common with hydrogen SIBO, and constipation is present with methane SIBO. Hydrogen sulfide SIBO is another form that feeds on sulfur rich foods. This produces rotten egg smelling gas.

There are many causes and contributing factors to the development of SIBO. A common cause is disruption of the wave that cleans the small intestine; this wave is called the Migrating Motor Complex (MMC). The MMC occurs every 90–120 minutes between meals when the body has been fasting. It sweeps the small intestines clean of bacteria. The MMC will not fire when a person is eating frequent small meals. It should occur on average ten to twelve times a day in a healthy person. For someone with SIBO, however, it may happen only two to four times a day. Intestinal nerve damage from medications, infection, surgery, and diabetes can prevent the MMC from firing. Other causes of SIBO are food poisoning, slow motility caused by low thyroid, neurotransmitter imbalance, autoimmune conditions, parasites and protozoa, alcohol consumption, valve dysfunction, obstructions, adhesions, vagus nerve damage, and insufficient digestive enzymes.

The SIBO gas travels a long time before leaving the body. Much of these gases are absorbed. When detoxification pathways are not working optimally, gases can cause nausea, skin issues, migraines, fatigue, mood swings, joint pain, and brain fog. Repairing detoxification needs to be done first, as killing pathogens will only release more gases and toxins.

Testing is done via breath test or endoscopy. The problem with endoscopy is it checks only the first part of the small intestine. It is also invasive and expensive. A breath test with lactulose, where sampling is done every twenty minutes for two hours, gives a complete picture of the entire small intestine. It takes two hours for the lactulose to travel through the small intestine. Testing will show the severity and type(s) of gas. Hydrogen sulfide SIBO will show as a negative SIBO test, as the hydrogen sulfide producing bacteria will consume the methane and hydrogen gas. Since we do not see hydrogen sulfide SIBO on a breath test, one can determine whether they have it if they have a sulfur sensitivity and experience gas that smells like rotten eggs after eating sulfur foods.

Test preparation is key when testing for SIBO. I have seen some inadequate test preparation, and it is no wonder there are many false negatives. For seven days prior to testing, stop taking all antimicrobials, flushes, enemas, probiotics, and binders. Twenty-four hours prior to testing, consume only meat, oils, eggs, water, salt, pepper, and jasmine rice. Nothing else. Fast for twelve hours before testing, then follow the instructions on the test kit. People who are diabetic or lactulose intolerant should discuss other testing options with their practitioner. If constipation is present, the test preparation should be done for two days prior to testing. See your practitioner for test results.

Antibiotics are often prescribed for a positive test result. Usually Rifaximin, Neomycin, Flagyl, or Metronidazole are chosen. Personally, I would never take these, as I have seen severe, long-term injury happen too many times. It is akin to playing Russian Roulette. The possible injury is much worse than the symptoms of SIBO. By first addressing detoxification and supporting the body, most symptoms will disappear. A natural remedy is safer, in my opinion.

A low FODMAP diet or the Specific Carbohydrate Diet does not clear up SIBO, it only causes it to go dormant. It will come back when a person introduces food, and for most people, these diets are not sustainable long term. During a SIBO protocol, these diets should not be followed, as the dormant bacteria will not be touched by the antimicrobials. It is better to feed SIBO while doing a protocol. After a protocol is complete, a low FODMAP diet or SCD for three months is used before reintroducing foods.

Natural options for SIBO are berberine, neem, oregano, allicin (found in garlic, but do not use garlic), lauric acid (from coconut), and enteric-coated peppermint oil. Methane SIBO does best with allicin, but allicin is contraindicated for people with hydrogen sulfide SIBO or issues with sulfur. Some great products are FC Cidal, Lauricidin, Dysbiocide, Candibactin, Ayush Neem Plus, Dr. Whitaker's Berberine, ADP, Silvercillin, and Atrantil. Biofilm busters can be used, but there are not enough studies to show if they are effective or even necessary. Prebiotics can be used during a protocol to help feed SIBO so it can be better targeted by antimicrobials. Do not use prebiotics before or after your protocol.

For hydrogen sulfide SIBO, reducing sulfur and working on detoxification is key. Personally, I healed from hydrogen sulfide SIBO. Though I can eat sulfur foods, I do so in moderation.

Most probiotics will feed SIBO. SIBO is good bacteria in the wrong place. Safe forms of probiotics include Megaspore and other spore-based and soil-based probiotics, L. casei, L. plantarum, L. johnsonii, Streptococcus faecalis, B. brevis, B. infantis, and B. lactis. Avoid D lactate forms (acidophilus being one of them, which is in most brands of probiotics). Prebiotics will feed SIBO and include FOS, MOS, GOS, inulin, and arabinogalactan.

Retesting should be done within two weeks of a natural protocol. The ideal is lower levels of gases or the gases being gone on the retest. If the levels are lower, another round can be done. It they are gone, a low FODMAP diet for three months is the next step. After a protocol is complete and gases are gone, adding a prokinetic to speed up transit time and eating three meals per day helps with the MMC. A prokinetic can be used for three months, though for some it may be needed up to a year or longer, depending on the cause of SIBO. If nerve damage is the cause, prokinetics may be needed long-term. Iberogast, ginger,

D. limonene, and Motil Pro are all great options. There are many low FODMAP and SCD diet plans in various books and online.

Root Causes of Symptoms

This section will go over the most common symptoms I encounter and their most common root causes.

Anxiety

Anxiety is one of the most common symptoms reported by clients. The most common root causes of anxiety are neurotransmitter imbalance, adrenal dysfunction, hormone imbalance, and toxin overload. Anxiety needs to be addressed first, as the body cannot heal if it is in fight or flight mode. Run genetics and Organic Acids Test to understand one's breakdown of serotonin, dopamine, and GABA, then get precursors and cofactors up. Work on detoxification pathways so the body can remove toxins properly and safely from the body, without affecting the brain. Mindset training is of utmost importance, as you will learn to recognize and change dysfunctional thought patterns. Next, run a DUTCH Test and support hormones and adrenals. See the corresponding sections on each of those systems.

Depression

The most common root causes of depression are neurotransmitter imbalance, hormone imbalance, thyroid dysfunction, and mindset. First of all, run a genetics and Organic Acids Test and balance neurotransmitters. Use mindset work to address emotional traumas, guilt, and existential crises like lack of passion and purpose. The opposite of depression is expression. Too often we are suppressing an emotion that needs to be expressed. After this, run a DUTCH Test and support sex hormones. See the corresponding sections on each of those systems in the "Appendix."

Insomnia

The root causes of insomnia are neurotransmitter imbalance, hormone imbalance, adrenal dysfunction, dysfunctional circadian rhythms, detoxification issues, pathogens, and uncontrolled thoughts. Run genetics and Organic Acids Test to balance neurotransmitters. Serotonin is a building block of melatonin; when serotonin is low, you cannot make melatonin. Melatonin is needed to sleep. It is best to test before supplementing with melatonin, as people tend to take way more than is needed, and sometimes low melatonin is not even the problem. Taking too much of any supplement to turn off thoughts so you can sleep is going below thought. When thoughts are an issue, mindset training must be implemented. It is important to learn meditation and breathing techniques to put the body into a state of relaxation. If my thoughts are racing, I will turn on a mindset book like the *Tao Te Ching* or something by Eckhart Tolle. His relaxing voice helps me get to sleep.

Low GABA can contribute to the inability to fall asleep and contribute to racing thoughts. High cortisol levels can also provide the second wind at night and prevent sleep. Additionally, cortisol can spike during the night in response to detoxification and pathogens. The body likes to detoxify between 2:00 a.m. and 4:00 a.m., which can cause a person to wake up and have issues going back to sleep. Though we can lower cortisol, we want to address and support detoxification pathways. Pathogens are more active at night, and an immune response to deal with the more active pathogens can also spike cortisol and cause a person to awaken. Gut work will help if this is the case. Sometimes people do not start to sleep well until their pathogen load has been decreased. Sleep mindset is important for people whose sleep issues are caused by detoxification issues or pathogens, as it will take time for it to improve. Learning to not get angry, frustrated, or anxious about not sleeping and how they feel the next day will allow the body to stay calm. Any negative emotions will add fuel to the fire by causing an even bigger stress response.

Circadian rhythm dysfunction is a real issue with sleep and can be a challenge for people to address. When you are unable to sleep for a few nights in a row, the tendency is to sleep in the next morning. Waking up late throws off the cortisol curve, causing cortisol to drop in morning and spike at night. It is a vicious cycle. The way to end it is with adjusting the time you wake up, not your bedtime. Adjusting wake up time should be done gradually. Rarely do I see an abrupt cold turkey change be successful in the long-term when it comes to sleep or diet. If you wake up at 12:00 p.m. every day, set your wake time to thirty minutes earlier each week, regardless of what time you go to bed. The commitment to the new wake up time is vital. Slow and steady changes work.

Likewise, practicing a good bedtime routine is important. The brain likes habits, so do the same thing each night before bed to prepare your brain for sleep. Turn off all technology that emits blue light two hours before bedtime. Have a nice bath, brush your teeth, read, meditate, and then go to bed. If sleep does not happen, turn on a meditation or an audiobook. If you still do not end up sleeping, you can spend your nights doing mindset training.

Ideal wake up times are between 6:00 a.m. and 8:00 a.m. Some people like the 5:00 a.m. club, and there is a push for the most successful people being up at 5:00 a.m. To me, it really does not matter. I wake up around 8:00 a.m. every day, depending on when Kaiden awakens, as we co-sleep. I feel I am super focused, successful, fulfilled, and full of joy. If 5:00 a.m. really feels terrible to you, and you dread it, do not do it just to fit in with the cool kids.

IC and Chronic Vaginal Issues

What I have found to be the root causes of both these issues are oxalates, ammonia, sulfur, histamine, sex hormones, and biofilm infections. I start by running an Organic Acids Test to check oxalate and ammonia levels, and then genetics testing to determine predisposition to higher ammonia or sulfur issues. Once those issues are addressed, I run a DUTCH Test to check sex hormones and eventually work to clear pathogens. It is often the case that oxalates and ammonia appear low on the Organic Acids Test until detoxification support is started. CBS and MTHFR A1298C are both genetic mutations that increase ammonia. Lyme, Prevotella and H. pylori all contribute to higher ammonia levels. Sulfur sensitivity goes hand in hand with high oxalates and ammonia. It is often never a single issue causing the symptoms in the bladder and/or vagina but a combination of the above. Running a DUTCH Test is important, as any imbalance in sex hormones can affect the bladder lining and vaginal mucosa and flora. Many people think it is just high estrogen and mast cell issues that are the problem, but low estrogen, low progesterone, and high progesterone can also cause issues. Balance is key. People often try to guess at which hormones are imbalanced and take high amounts of DIM (Diindolylmethane) and I3C (indole 3 carbanol) to lower estrogen. This can cause more damage if low estrogen is affecting the vaginal or bladder lining and mucosa; it can compound the issue further if the bladder and vaginal issues are caused by oxalates and/or sulfur issues. Hydrogen sulfide SIBO with the signature rotten egg smell after eating foods high in sulfur can also increase sulfur and ammonia levels, making the person sensitive to it. When I eat too much sulfur, I start to smell the ammonia in my urine. If I ignore it, I will start smelling it in my vagina and in my body odor. If I keep on ignoring it and continue to eat high sulfur foods, it will cause bladder pain.

The effects of the sulfur were difficult to recognize. The effects from a high sulfur diet were not instantaneous but instead due to the accumulation. After I stopped eating the foods and increased detoxification support, it did not clear up instantly. This was another reason it took some time for me to figure it out. If sulfur is the cause, it takes time to detoxify. Mindset is important as it is likely that the person will feel better for a bit and then flare again. Over time, they will have less and less intense flares, and the flares will lessen in duration and frequency.

If histamine is contributing to the vaginal and bladder symptoms, it will usually respond to an antihistamine. If this is the case, results can take longer to achieve. I have found the key to healing from histamine issues is to remove the external and internal stress from the body. This includes getting support on board for the body by addressing deficiencies, repairing detoxification, systematically addressing pathogens in the gut, removing emotional stress, and removing heavy metals. Often people who have histamine issues do not see results until after gut work. It does not mean gut work should be done first to get results faster, as that is rarely successful.

Lastly, biofilm infections can affect both the bladder and the vagina. PCR testing is best to determine what is present. I have found that the vagina and bladder will clear up as the pathogens are addressed in the gut.

In my experience, many women who suffer from bladder or vaginal issues have a history of sexual abuse. Working through this emotional trauma is essential to healing. I found with myself that my issues were ninety-five percent resolved by addressing the physical issues, but there was still irritation after sex until I dealt with the emotional trauma.

Fatigue

Fatigue is another common symptom, and too often the focus is on the thyroid and adrenals. That is never my starting point. The most important things to look at are neurotransmitter balance, mitochondria, and plain old nutrient deficiencies. The Organic Acids Test and genetics test will give us great information on all three of these. If your body cannot make ATP, you are going to be tired (see "Organic Acids Test Analysis" section in the "Appendix" for mitochondrial support). If your brain is imbalanced, you are going to be tired. If you are in a state of anxiety or depression due to neurotransmitter imbalance, you are going to be tired. Imagine being chased by a tiger all day, every day. That is what anxiety does to you. Next is detoxification. If you are full of toxins, you are going to be tired. They have a huge impact on the brain and are largely responsible for brain fog.

Most of the time, people are told to follow an elimination diet when fatigue is present. These elimination diets cause further damage by increasing deficiencies, putting neurotransmitters further out of balance, increasing stress on the body, and depriving the body of fuel, which leads to more mitochondrial dysfunction. Most people feel worse on these diets but continue because they have been told certain foods are bad. Not getting your ideal fuel is another cause of chronic fatigue. The key is listening to your body, not a diet.

After neurotransmitters, detoxification, mitochondria, diet, and nutrient deficiency support are in place, it is time to look at sex hormones and adrenals. Both of these can contribute to fatigue. Too little free cortisol and low or high hormones can cause fatigue. The thyroid, of course, can cause fatigue, but I do not like to address it right away, unless antibodies are high and reverse T3 is under 15 ng/dL. Poor sleep and circadian rhythm dysfunction will play a role in fatigue, as well.

Last but not least is existential crisis. If the person is in a dead-end job, always on the go, not doing any self-care, and not fulfilling passion and purpose, then fatigue can be a symptom.

Fatigue really shows the importance of proper testing. There are too many variables and options to guess what is causing the fatigue. It also shows why it is so important to have a truly holistic approach. There usually are multiple causes for symptoms. Being systematic and addressing everything in sequence is best for covering all your bases.

When addressing fatigue, energy tends to return gradually. As energy returns, it is important not to expend it all trying to catch up on day-to-day tasks that were missed due to the fatigue. Energy must be conserved for gut work as clearing pathogens is stressful on the body. Time will allow for those stores to rebuild.

Weight Gain

Many people get frustrated that they struggle to lose weight. If people are adhering to diet and exercise changes that simply are not working, feelings of guilt and shame often occur because the weight refuses to come off. That, on top of society's fat shaming, can cause a lot of depression and anxiety. People will tell them they "are not trying hard enough," and they need to "just put down the food," when in reality, weight gain is no different than any other symptom. Weight gain or the inability to lose weight is a symptom of dysfunction. The first thing people do when they want to lose weight is cut calories. This is counterproductive. If it does work in the short-term, as soon as the person stops the calorie restriction, the weight will come back. The body, sensing the lack of food, increases fat storage.

Diet alone is not the answer and can often do more harm than good. Fueling the body is a must to lose weight. The focus should be on getting in a lot of micronutrients and sticking to whole foods. Grain should be consumed in moderation. A full thyroid panel is important. Often, people believe weight gain is due to the thyroid. It does play a big role, but usually, rT3 is elevated. This elevation will prevent NDT from working. It is possible to use T3 only to flush the rT3, but I prefer not to do that at the beginning. Our focus needs to be away from the symptoms and onto the root causes. If rT3 is not elevated, NDT can be used. When a person sees that their thyroid is outside of optimal ranges, it can help them get a sense of justification and let go of the blame and guilt.

So often people are trying to lose weight and doing everything right with their diet and exercise, but the body is storing fat because in the fat are toxins it cannot detoxify properly. To prevent the toxins from doing damage, the body stores them in the fat. It is a good survival mechanism. The body is always doing the best it can with the tools it has and finding love and gratitude for the body helps with body image and self-love. Having a positive body image and loving oneself moves the person into a healing state. Once the body is able to detoxify properly, it often begins to let go of the fat. Sex hormones and mitochondria are important to address if weight gain or the inability to lose weight is a symptom.

Candida and Chronic Yeast Infections

After a person takes antibiotics, yeast can overgrow. Because we see the yeast, we tend to blame it for our symptoms. I find this is seldom the cause and focusing on the yeast is rarely successful. Antibiotics are the straw that broke the camel's back. They affect good flora levels and can allow other pathogens or opportunistic microbes to take hold. Antibiotics are also hard on the liver and can cause gene mutations to become active. Many antibiotics can damage the vagus nerve and mitochondria. In general, they weaken the entire body.

I am not against antibiotics. There is a need for them. They save lives. Would you rather be dead or cleaning up the mess of an antibiotic? I would rather clean up the mess. I always first try to address a bacterial infection with natural remedies. Grapefruit seed extract, oil of oregano and olive leaf are my first choices. If there is no success within a couple days or symptoms get worse, it is time for an antibiotic. The body will be weakened not only from the antibiotic but from the infection itself. The focus needs to be on getting the body strong enough again to keep the yeast in check. When a yeast infection keeps coming back after antifungals, whether natural or not, it is a sign that a different approach is needed.

I have found success rebuilding the body, repairing detoxification, and then addressing the other pathogens that have taken hold, starting with parasites and protozoa, then bacteria, and finally, yeast. If yeast markers are very high on an Organic Acids Test, then I will add in some yeast support such as undecylenic acid. I have found the more often people have used antifungals, the more resistant their infections become, and the weaker their bodies get due to the toxicity of the medications. It is always good to test genetics for CYP mutations, as people with these mutations, along with other genes in methylation, have an increased chance of reacting adversely to medication.

Skin Issues

Skin issues include hives, rashes, acne, rosacea, and eczema. I have found the most common cause of skin issues to be dysfunction in detoxification. This can be in phase one, two or three pathways or a combination of them. Addressing detoxification pathways is always the first place I start for skin issues. Overall deficiencies can cause issues, as can sex hormone imbalance. The most common hormone imbalances affecting skin are low estrogen, high testosterone, high alpha testosterone metabolites, and androgen sensitivity.

If general histamine dysfunction is affecting the skin, it can take longer to clear up, as histamine response often does not tone down until the overall stress on the body is lowered by addressing pathogens, metals, emotional stress, and toxins.

Chronic infections of the skin clear up after gut work. When you rebalance bacteria in the gut, it affects the skin, as well. Mindset is needed to find self-love for the body that is doing the best it can with the tools it has, as the journey can be longer for some. Personally, I do not use soap on my skin, with the exception of my hands. This allows the bacteria balance to be undisturbed and the natural oils to be protected. For the harsh winters, I use jojoba oil, as it is close to the skin's natural sebum. I also rarely wear make-up, and if I do, I use a mineral powder. I do not use any other products on my skin. No matter how itchy, do not scratch. Scratching will increase the chance of infection and slow healing.

Headaches and Migraines

It is best to separate the root causes into internal and external causes. The external causes will be physical stress, injury, tension, poor posture, and eye strain due to screen time. In today's world, too much screen time should always be ruled out first. I personally do short durations at my computer with frequent breaks. I keep my computer and my phone at eye level and have no social media on my phone. For injuries and tension, use a heating pad on the neck and shoulders nightly for twenty minutes, take hot baths, and do self-massage. Massage therapists, physiotherapists, chiropractors, osteopaths, and acupuncturists also help.

For internal root causes, I have found the most common cause to be a neurotransmitter imbalance, in particular, low serotonin. Second would be issues with dctoxification. Hormone imbalance comes in third. See corresponding sections on those issues.

Lyme, Mold, and Chronic Viral Infections

I grouped these together because it seems that everyone who comes to me believes they have Lyme and mold. I am not downplaying either. I see a trend where practitioners label people with both of these and proceed to cause more harm than good. Chronic Lyme is usually treated with multiple rounds of antibiotics or very intense herbal protocols. Mold is usually treated with toxic binders. I have seen both routes do a lot of damage.

For mold, the first step is for a person to confirm they have mold in their house, workplace, or vehicle, not their body. Almost every mycotoxin test I have run on people comes back with elevated levels. The truth is, there is mold everywhere. It is good to see that your body is actively detoxifying it. If there are high levels in the home, it is important to move or remediate the mold. Once that is done, detoxification pathways first need to be repaired, and the body needs to be supported. Then, gentle binders can be added in to help remove the mold. I grew up in mold. I was very sensitive to mold until I repaired my detoxification pathways. Though it no longer causes issues for me, I choose to live in as clean of an environment as possible.

For Lyme, my approach is the same. Work on supporting the body and repairing detoxification pathways. Once the body is supported, work on parasites and protozoa and their biofilm. Lyme hides in their biofilm, which keeps it safe from being destroyed by antibiotics or herbal treatments. It is counterproductive to try to address Lyme bacteria until the biofilm of these pathogens is addressed. It just weakens the body, destroys good flora, and creates resistance.

For viruses: unless the virus has reactivated, it is best to focus on rebuilding, rebalancing, and repairing the body while removing external and internal stress, so that the body is able to keep viruses in check on its own. I do not believe chronic viral infections are the root cause of all illness. They are just another internal stressor.

Joint Pain, Muscle Pain, Tingling, and Numbness

The most common internal cause of pain in the joints and muscles will be toxin overload and oxalates. Working on detoxification pathways brings the most relief, as does toning down overall inflammation by reducing stress on the body. See corresponding sections on those areas.

Though issues with detoxification can cause pain, tingling, and numbness, more often than not muscle tension is responsible for them. Joint pain is often a trigger point in a muscle referring to a joint. For example, I always thought I had knee issues. As a massage therapist, I learned the trigger points that refer to the knee. When I addressed mine, my knee pain went away. For me, my glutes and iliotibial band are the most common causes. In the five years I practiced as a massage therapist, I saw this time and time again working with thousands of people. Their joint pain would go away with massaging, stretching, and heating the muscles. Tight muscles are also the most common cause of tingling and numbness, as they impinge on nerves.

The Mind-Body Connection

Our society has programed us to believe that symptoms mean something serious is wrong with us. The fear that comes with thinking you have a serious illness breaks down the body. I believe I created my illness this way. I was convinced I had a serious illness, and all my focus was on it. Through my journey, I learned how my fear and thoughts brought me to seeking a diagnosis label. The label itself was just a mashup of symptoms that all had their own root causes. The migraines and depression were caused by imbalances in my brain and issues with detoxification; the joint pain was caused by tight muscles and trigger points; and the IC was caused by oxalate and ammonia overload.

In "Part One: Body," I went over my whole-body approach to healing. Phase One involved rebuilding, rebalancing, and repairing the body. We started by getting a foundation support in place using the Organic Acids Test, genetics test, blood test and DUTCH Test, while working toward a balanced, whole food diet. These tests addressed neurotransmitters, the thyroid, hormones, deficiencies, adrenals, mitochondria, and detoxification pathways. Phase Two moved to removing stress by addressing pathogens with gut work and heavy metal detoxification. Now, we will shift our focus to the mind and how we can stop using our thoughts to create illness, and instead use them to help heal.

PART TWO

MIND

The Importance of Meditation, Mindfulness, and Mindset Training

Everything is energy. All energy has a frequency, a vibration. White light is made up of the rainbow of colors, red with the lowest frequency and violet with the highest. Humans are made of matter, which is made of energy. If we take the most powerful microscopes and zoom in on any cell in the body, we go past the cells, DNA, base molecules, atoms, and electrons all the way down to quanta of energy and a lot of space. What is mind-blowing at this quantum level is that the act of observing these subatomic particles changes how they behave! It is as though they are aware of us and make decisions. In order to better understand this principle, take a second to look up the double-slit experiment and observer effect on the internet. All of us are made up mostly of space and these quanta of energy. When we put these quanta through a particle accelerator, they disappear and reappear out of nothingness. At this level, there is no time and no boundaries. This "no-thing"-ness is the universal consciousness, where all matter, all beings, and the universe itself originated. We are connected to it. Our thoughts themselves cannot be found. They, too, are believed to come from this quantum field. When we quiet the mind and become the observer, our thoughts seem to behave just like quanta, randomly coming from nowhere. Voices not heard in years, memories from childhood that have never been thought of, and ideas and inspiration that could never have been imagined.

We, too, have an electromagnetic energy. Our bodies thrive when we are vibrating at a higher frequency. Our thoughts are energy and create our emotions. Our emotions are energy. Our thoughts and emotions determine our bodies' vibrations. Emotions of joy, love, gratitude, passion, enthusiasm, and happiness are high vibrations. Frustration, impatience, disappointment, doubt, worry, anger, jealousy, revenge, guilt, fear, and depression are low vibrations. You can determine your vibration by how you feel. There is no need to monitor each thought, though you can learn how to use your thoughts to create a higher vibration and to raise your consciousness level.

Meditation, mindfulness, and mindset training are all tools essential to shifting a person's vibration from lower to higher frequencies. Each one is different, yet the terms can be used interchangeably. Meditation is the act of becoming aware of one's thoughts, body, and environment. Mindfulness is the practice of becoming present in the moment. It is a form of meditation and can be used anytime to tune in to the observer. Mindset training includes any techniques to strengthen the mind and gain mastery of oneself. Both mindfulness and meditation can be included under mindset training. Since "meditation" is often associated with sitting down for an intended period of time, I will use this definition throughout the book. Though I will cover the benefits of meditation here, the meditations themselves are in "Part Three: Spirit." I will use the word "mindfulness" to mean becoming the observer in the moment, not an intentional practice but a way of stepping back outside yourself at any moment during the day. I will use the term "mindset training" to include any technique used for training the mind. All three are used to relax the body and stop the flight or fight response. With practice in meditation, mindfulness, and mindset training, a person is enabled to dissociate from pain and other symptoms. Meditation and mindset training also raise vibrations through specific visualizations that activate the Laws of Attraction. Through meditation and mindfulness, we connect with our higher selves and to universal consciousness.

My goal as a health coach is to give my clients the tools they need to heal their bodies from chronic illness and get to an optimal state of health. In "Part One: Body," I outlined the process of how to rebuild the body by addressing imbalances and deficiencies, repairing detoxification pathways, and removing stress. I use functional labs to determine what the body needs to heal itself. I do not look for illness. Looking for illness only creates more of it and puts a label on the body. Instead, I look for healing opportunities. The body wants to return to health. Healing is the body's only goal; it just needs the tools to do so. We provide the body with the tools through whole foods, supplements, and herbs.

For the body to have any chance at success in healing itself, a person must shift their vibration from a lower frequency to a higher one. Most people with chronic illness are in a state of depression, anxiety, anger, or hopelessness. Healing the mind and spirit are just as important to overcoming chronic illness as addressing the physical issues. Of the hundreds of clients I have worked with, the ones that put the effort into mindset and spiritual growth get the best results. Those who put no effort into mindset get the lowest results. I have had clients come to me with chronic pain, rashes all over their bodies, and severe anxiety. They have done only mindset training and cleared up those issues without any supplements or herbs. There are stories from all over the world of spontaneous remission from every illness through a shift in consciousness. *Anatomy of an Illness* by Norman Cousins and *Dying to Be Me* by Anita Moorjani are great books that illustrate this.

When healing, we also want to remove external stress. Most people think this means disengaging from all emotional stress in life by staying away from toxic people, changing jobs, and changing relationships. While this may be necessary in some instances for a time, we want to gain tools to handle stress in life. We want to change how we respond to stress so that stressful events turn into "just" events. The tools I share in this book are to help you shift your vibration to peace and joy so you can heal your body. The healing journey is not linear, and for some people it can take time, especially those who have been injured by medication. The healing journey does not go better, better, better, best. There are ups and downs. The good days become more frequent, but the not-so-good days will still be there. In time, they become fewer and fewer. Meditation and other mindset training tools will make the journey peaceful. It prevents a spiral of negativity when the not-so-good days occur. This allows those not-so-good days to pass more quickly.

Releasing Blocks to Mindset Training

The biggest block people have toward doing mindset training is the perception that if they admit their mind has any power, then that must mean everything they are experiencing is all in their head. Many people who suffer from chronic illness do not have a disease diagnosis. They go from doctor to doctor, telling them that something is wrong, yet all tests come back normal. The doctor will blame it on anxiety or depression, saying, "It is all in your head. Here is an antidepressant or anti-anxiety medication to turn off that symptom." This makes them feel that they are crazy because of the huge stigma behind mental health issues.

When someone is then told to work on their mindset, a block comes up immediately. Defenses are raised to protect themselves from a label. Had the doctor explained that their thoughts have powerful effects on their body and cause a physiological response, and that their negative thoughts break down the body and cause illness, there would be no resistance. Had the doctor explained that, through training, they could learn to change their thought patterns and even rise above thought, a lot less medication would be prescribed, and our world would be a healthier, happier, more peaceful place. Why don't they? First, doctors are not trained that way. The pharmaceutical industry profits from people being on medication. Anti-anxiety and antidepressant medications go below thought to sedate the mind. Also, much of society wants a quick fix, so there is a large market for quick fixes. At the end of the day, responsibility falls on the individual to become educated on their different options. Healing requires us to take responsibility for all the choices we have made in our lives, which can be a hard pill to swallow. Taking responsibility for everything that happens in your life or has happened is one of the most challenging aspects of spiritual development. Taking responsibility is the common theme in all of the books I have read on self-growth. Because of this, it is best to get started with it and address any blocks that come up right away.

When people hear they are responsible for everything in their life and that they have either attracted, created, or allowed every event to happen, it either empowers them or it triggers a lot of anger, shame, and guilt. We are responsible for most things in our lives if we dig deep and look at the entire situation. Many spiritual teachers believe we are responsible for all things that happen to us. That is hard for many people to come to terms with. How does a person attract rape, a childhood disease, a car accident, or an act of nature? There are cases like these where it is tough to see the correlation, and sometimes you may not be able to see it at all.

When I first heard this, I believed it applied to most things but not to everything. What got me was how could a child whose brain is not yet formed and is not conscious, attract a serious childhood illness or even death? Now I have come to believe we choose to be here, and before we come into this life, we choose our parents and the circumstances we will experience. I believe there are some very wise souls who come into this world knowing they may experience things like cancer or other illness at a very young age in order to teach love, compassion, and other lessons. This belief brings me peace on my journey. It is up to you to create beliefs that serve you. If you are unable to believe that you created or allowed everything in your life, that is okay. However, we want to believe that right now we are responsible for *how we react* to our pasts and we are responsible for *how we respond* to current and future events. There cannot be any doubt there. You get to choose how you respond now. You have a choice. By taking responsibility, it allows us to empower ourselves and create our futures.

We are also conditioned as a society to blame others. When we come face to face with responsibility, that blame then ends up being redirected onto oneself. This does not feel good. It is totally normal if this happens. It is much easier to blame others than take responsibility. As an adult, I had choices. I chose to keep eating terribly, stressed myself out, took medications, and spent way too much time playing video games. It was easy to see how I attracted the illness, not only by not taking care of my body but also by the thoughts I was thinking and my emotional state. I was not a very happy person unless my environment was making me happy; I was always looking for external happiness. It hurt when I took responsibility because all I knew was how to blame.

Blame is not responsibility. Blaming is giving away your power. Responsibility is realizing that I did the best with the tools, knowledge, skills, and level of consciousness I had at the time. That goes for everyone, everywhere. My past was exactly what I needed to go through to get to where I am today. I take responsibility for it, as I also had the choice to learn new tools. At that time, I was unconscious and unaware of the effects my thoughts and actions were having on creating my life. Now I am conscious and aware, and now I can make changes. Now I can choose to learn and grow.

The most important tool to learn is that your response is where your power lies; the event itself is neutral. Your response is your thoughts, beliefs, and actions. Our thoughts create our beliefs; how we think will determine our actions. The actions we take will determine the outcome. Through mindset training, we connect with our higher selves and can therefore choose a response that will create the best outcome. An outer-directed person believes that events cause a problem and something outside of them will fix it. An inner-directed person takes responsibility for what happens without guilt, shame, or feelings of failure. They recognize mistakes occur as part of the learning process and grow from them. They know they can solve whatever comes their way. If you were not born an inner-directed person, that's okay. I definitely was not born an inner-directed person.

Exercise #1: Taking Responsibility: When something fails to turn out the way you want it, ask: "How did I create or allow this? How can I respond differently next time?"

We do not want to change just our response to events; it is also important to change our beliefs around events to ones that serve us and create peace. Accepting reality creates peace. No amount of anger or sadness about things we believe should not have happened will ever change the past. "When we argue with reality we lose, only one hundred percent of the time," is one of my favorite Byron Katie quotes. Every should or should not is an argument with reality. We will still feel anger or sadness when things happen in life. Taking responsibility is learning to not get stuck there and be defined by the things that happen to us. By changing our beliefs and our response to events, we can use them to fuel our growth and take our power back.

Mindset training is the best way to take our power back, as we can use it to harness the power of our thoughts. It requires dedication, time, focus, and energy. We will now look at the science behind how our thoughts affect the body, so we can understand that power.

Understanding the Cortisol Response

Close your eyes and imagine yourself at the top of the highest building you have ever seen. The CNN Tower, the Sky Tower, the Skylon, or even a tall apartment building will work. See yourself on the roof. Walk toward the edge. There are no railings to hold you in. You are so high up that the wind is causing you to sway. As you get closer to the edge of the tower, you can see the traffic below. The people are so small they look like ants. You walk closer to the edge and look down at your feet. You carefully put the toes of a foot over. Just then, a gust of wind hits you and you fall off the edge. Thankfully, your friend grabs your arm and pulls you to safety. Come back to your body and feel the safety of your feet on the ground.

The first time I did that visualization, I was at Jack Canfield's *Breakthrough to Success* seminar. Most of the participants reported the following sensations from doing the visualization: sweating, shaking, nausea, weakness, a sudden jump reflex as they felt they were falling, swaying, rapid heart rate, and anxiety. But all the while, they were sitting safely in a chair. The same happens when we read a horror novel, and we have all had that dream where we fall off an edge and jerk awake, heart pounding, sweating, feeling sick to our stomachs, knowing there is no way we will fall asleep anytime soon. That is the stress response. That is how powerful your thoughts are.

The cortisol, aka, stress response is a powerful, real, measured, biological event in the body. In the normal stress response, the amygdala in the brain senses a threat and tells the hypothalamus to activate the sympathetic nervous system. It sends signals to the adrenal glands to produce epinephrine and adrenaline. Heart rate, pulse, and blood pressure increase to move nutrients to the muscles. Stores of glucose are released to fuel the body. If the threat continues, the brain signals the adrenal glands to pump out cortisol, allowing the body to stay in fight or flight mode. Digestion slows. Who needs to digest food when running from a tiger? When the threat passes, the levels of cortisol fall, and the parasympathetic nervous system (which is responsible for rest, repair, and digestion) takes over. The stress response is meant to happen occasionally in response to a true threat on the body.

Most people in the world walk around all day thinking the same stressful thoughts over and over: not having enough money, not having the body they want, not having the relationship they want, climate change, getting sick and dying, viruses killing them or their family, etc. We as a species are stuck in a chronic fear cycle. This, of course, is perpetuated by the media. Most of what we see on the news is negative: murders, viral pandemics, floods, hurricanes, stock market crashes, charged political views, and so much more. It is not surprising, as they are largely funded by an industry that profits from people being sick. Count the number of ads you see in a day for medications. Not sleeping? Depressed? Have anxiety? It is no wonder when you look at where our thoughts are. Do not worry, there is a pill for that. I am not against medicine. I have a huge respect for emergency medicine; however, I prefer a different approach for chronic illness.

Personally, I stopped watching the news many years ago and have also turned off social media except for work-related purposes. Many people in the world are currently so afraid of dying that they have stopped living. Remember, the body does not know the difference between a thought and a real event. When you imagine yourself or your family dying, the body believes it is just as serious as being chased by a tiger in real life. An imagined threat from the untrained mind is as powerful as a real-life threat.

The body is not meant to be in a chronic state of flight or fight. When the stress response happens frequently or, for many people, almost nonstop all day, the body is always in a state of breakdown. Long-term effects include dysfunctions in immune activity like decreased secretory IgA (a first line of immune defense in the gastrointestinal tract), increased circulating IgG (causes immune reactions to non-harmful substances like food), decreased natural killer-cell function (needed to prevent cancer), and decreased lymphocytes (needed to fight viruses and bacteria). Chronically high cortisol also leads to an increase in bone loss, as nutrients are metabolized to fuel the body for the perceived threat. This also causes increased fat accumulation as the body tries to build stores to handle the ongoing threat, muscle breakdown, insulin sensitivity, and decreased sex hormone levels as reserves are depleted. You will not need to reproduce when running from a tiger nonstop all day. It is no wonder we see so much hormone imbalance today. The cofactors needed to create neurotransmitters also become depleted, which creates a vicious cycle. No serotonin or GABA means more anxiety and depression. The entire body is affected by chronic stress.

It is important to balance and support neurotransmitters, sex hormones, and adrenal glands with supplements and herbs, as they all play a large role in the stress response and easily have their stores taxed when the body is under chronic stress. We want to immediately start supporting the body so it can begin to heal. That is why I begin by running tests to see what these systems need while beginning mindset training, as it is also essential to change the thought patterns. Supplements may help you be in a calmer, more positive state, but the work on the mind still needs to be done. There is no getting around it. It is amazing that when the mind is trained to no longer focus on the negative but to focus on the positive, the support the body needs decreases significantly. When the body is in the parasympathetic state, then rest, repair, and digestion can finally occur. Until then, you are just going to burn through any resources you give to the body. Stressful events in life will always happen. When you do the mindset training, the stressful events become "just" events. It may be necessary to disengage from work and stressful relationships, and you may need to get help until the body is sufficiently supported and mindset work has begun, but we can never remove the stress in our life forever. In order to heal and stay healthy, we must learn to change our responses to stressful events.

As you can see from the skyscraper demonstration, you do have the power to control your thoughts. Right now, you are more than likely stuck in reaction mode. An event happens and you react, there is no connection to your higher brain function, and you have not been able to separate yourself as the observer.

The Biology of the Brain

Some people are so entrenched in a repetitive negative thought pattern that they cannot hear their thoughts. When they think back to a time that they felt anxious, all they feel is the feeling of anxiety. The feeling is that powerful. Being stuck in a negative thought pattern and having patterns of reaction to stress are also a physiological response. We will now take a closer look into the functioning of the brain.

We have a higher or upper brain that is responsible for higher thinking called the prefrontal cortex. It is responsible for sound decision-making, planning, flexibility, adaptability, empathy, and morality. The lower brain is responsible for flight or fight. It is reactive.

The brain is always changing. It changes through experience. This is great, as it means we can learn new things and rewire the brain at any age. The upper brain is more evolved and can give you a fuller perspective on life. It allows you to see things clearly. It is sophisticated. From a biological perspective, the lower reactive brain is in total control, and there is no connection to higher brain function when people are reacting so strongly that they cannot differentiate their thoughts. When the amygdala and lower brain are fired, reasoning cannot happen. That is why telling someone to "calm down" never works. Integration allows the upper and lower brains to work together. Where attention goes, neurons fire and connections grow. The more you use new connections, the more the brain chooses those new connections. Integration creates more integration. The more we engage the upper brain in times of stress, the more fibers we grow from the upper brain to the lower brain. These fibers will strengthen and become the new response, rewriting the old patterns the more they are used. When a stressful event happens in the future, it will trigger these new pathways.

To learn these new skills, a person first needs to be in a calm state. This is where meditation and mindset training come in. The more you use these tools in a calm state, the more likely it is that you will use the tools in a mildly reactive state. The more you use these tools in a mildly reactive state, the more neural pathways are formed between the lower and upper areas of the brain and the more you will use them in a highly reactive state. They will become your new pattern because of those connections. Most people do not have a well-integrated brain, and their lower, reactive brain rules them. Like learning to play piano, practice is needed to develop and strengthen the new neural pathways. It is why mindset training needs to be a daily, repetitive practice.

The science behind post-traumatic stress is remarkable. Implicit memory is always recording. It is the only memory functioning from the time in the womb, and it is based on associations. For example, when you hear a song from your childhood you will suddenly remember something that happened while the song was playing. Explicit memories are those that we recall. Memory is not an accurate representation of what happened. Your mental state at the time of the memory and the time of recall will change your perception of it. This is why two people can have completely different memories of the same event. Since huge emotions can be stored in an implicit memory, when an implicit memory is triggered through something in the present, the emotions also arise. These emotions can be intense, causing the lower brain to take control. Since implicit memory is not something we can consciously recall on demand, it can take time to recognize what is triggering the intense emotions. Often, a third party is needed to make the connection and to help repair it. A good way to recognize an implicit memory being triggered as the cause of a negative emotion is if you respond in a big way to something that should not cause much stress.

Letting Go of Negative

For the rest of this book, I will try not to use the words "negative emotions" or "negative thoughts." The word "negative" has the connotation of "bad" for most people. There are no bad thoughts. The perceived negative thoughts have an important purpose. They tell you when you are not connected to your higher self. Events that are perceived to be negative also have a purpose. They create a contrast between what we want and what we do not want. We would not have anything to strive for if there were no negative events in the world. Expansion would stop. The perceived negative events can also be what is needed for great insight, spiritual growth, and change. More often than not, without a fall we would not have the momentum to make that next leap in our spiritual journey. The magnificence of the universe is in its infinite diversity. Beauty and meaning come through this diversity. According to Stephen Mitchell's translation of the second verse of the *Tao Te Ching*, "When people see some things as beautiful, other things become ugly, when people see some things as good, other things become bad, being and nonbeing create each other. Difficult and easy support each other. Long and short define each other." This contrast is at the core of all things in the universe.

Instead of using the term "negative" for thoughts of what we do not want and "negative" for emotions like anger, hate and frustration, I will use the phrase "lower frequency" or "lower vibration." The other reason I do not like the word "negative" when it comes to emotions is because it can create feelings of shame and guilt. "I know I should not be thinking that way," is something I hear often. There really are no shoulds and should nots. You are not bad for having lower-vibration emotions. They are part of self-growth. They are going to occur. It is a choice of whether or not you stay stuck with lower-vibration emotions. It is a choice to see them as a learning experience. It is a choice to focus on what you do want instead of what you do not want. At the end of the day, do you want to feel good? If you do have a sincere desire to feel good, then learning these tools will help you shift more easily and more quickly to higher-vibration states. Higher-vibration states are where healing occurs.

One of my favorite sayings from Wayne Dyer is, "When you squeeze an orange, orange juice comes out because that is what is inside the orange." When someone squeezes you, what comes out? Anger, hate, and fear, or love, patience, and kindness? Whatever is inside is going to come out. The person doing the squeezing is not what makes those things come out. I would like love, patience, and kindness to come out of me when I am put under pressure. I remind myself, "I can choose love; I can choose peace; I can choose compassion."

I say this to myself when I feel frustrated or upset, not because I feel that these are bad or because I get upset with myself. It is a spiritual aspiration I am working toward. When I feel love, peace, and compassion, I feel connected to source energy. The lower-frequency emotions are just a signpost that I have more work to do or there is something I need to express. They are not a judgment. Each judgment takes you away from your goal of peace. You only define yourself when you judge others and yourself. What you judge in others, you strengthen in yourself. All people are a mirror. We want to see where we judge others and ourselves. If you see something in someone else you do not like, it is because it is in you also. It is another cue to work on your doubts, fears, and self-love. A person's greatest weakness is also their greatest strength. Under numbness and unconsciousness is empowerment. From apathy comes caring. Under grief is great joy. From fear comes great faith. From anger comes responsibility and forgiveness. Beneath pain is great love. I love the quote from Ralph Waldo Emerson, "The whole course of things goes to teach us faith." Meditation and mindset training help us on our path.

The Laws of Attraction

Besides focusing on what we want in order to feel good, we also focus on what we want in order to activate the Laws of Attraction. The basis of the Laws of Attraction is "what you focus on, you get more of." Thoughts become things. If you are focusing on things that you do not like, you will attract into your life more things that cause you to feel the same way. When you focus on what you want and what makes you feel good, you will attract it and other things that make you feel good. The Laws of Attraction are always at work. It does not matter whether you are conscious of them or not, or even whether you believe in them. They are always working, just like gravity, and it does not take long experimenting with the Laws of Attraction to see how true this is. In the book *The Secret*, Rhonda Byrne gives many examples of how people were able to manifest objects exactly how they thought about them. One example that stands out for me was when I was first starting cross country jumping with my horse, Vala. She was terrified of the big blue barrels. She was just learning to jump, and they were quite big for her confidence level even though she is a very large horse. I had remembered seeing smaller barrels that I wanted to buy in order to train her. I called everywhere in town, and no one had any. I was so focused on those barrels. A few days later, I drove to my aunt's house, and there they were, sitting against her garage. Three small barrels, two blue and one green. I asked her where they came from, and she said her son had dropped them off. I called to ask him why he had brought them. He said he had decided to bring them there to be cleaned, out of the blue. I asked if I could have them, and he said yes. Coincidence? Maybe. I call it attraction and have seen too many so-called coincidences to not believe. The more you practice manifesting, the more you will see the synchronicity.

Often, I find resistance to the Laws of Attraction because people stuck in an anxious thought pattern will then have anxiety toward any negative thought they have. They will get into blame, shame, and resentment toward themselves. The Laws of Attraction are always happening, so whether the anxious person is aware of it or not does not matter. Whether they are focusing on anxiety toward life or toward their thoughts, there is no difference. The feeling of anxiety would be the same. They would still attract more to be anxious about, and they would still feel anxious. Feelings are what matter. At least by understanding how their thoughts affect their attraction point and create their lives, they are able to work on their thoughts instead of always focusing on changing external events. If they did not know their thoughts had consequences, they would never work to change them and would keep attracting more to be anxious about.

We can also look at the Laws of Attraction in another way to help reduce the anxiety around lower-vibration thoughts manifesting. For most people, thinking about something does not create an instantaneous response. It takes persistent thoughts of what we want to create in order to attract it. Are our thoughts enough? Sometimes, but usually, it is what our thoughts cause us to do that is key. When we think about what we want, we are motivated to take action and do things to get what we want. Also, thinking about what we want instead of focusing on things we perceive as negative and bad, shifts our vibration and energy. This allows us to see the world in a different light and choose better responses, so we get a better outcome. Fear is not bad. It is an essential survival instinct. Without it, we would not be here. Be grateful for your fears. They keep you safe. Through mindset training, we learn to recognize fears of the ego and work to become confident in our abilities to handle anything life brings our way. It is also important to remember that regardless of how positive we are, perceived negative events will happen in our lives. They are needed for growth and expansion.

The first step in shifting vibration is becoming aware of your thoughts and feelings. Everyone is on their own path, and the time it takes to shift to higher vibrational thought patterns is different for each individual. Regardless, it is still a good thing to shift from the outer, physical focus to an inward, spiritual focus. It is next to impossible to monitor every thought we have. Instead, use your feelings as your gauge. If you do not feel those higher-frequency emotions, then take a look at your thoughts. If you are always feeling anger, you will attract more things that make you angry. Low-vibration feelings and thoughts are much less powerful than high-vibration feelings and thoughts, which means you must think them a lot, over and over, for them to have the power to attract.

High-vibration thoughts and feelings are much more powerful and counterbalance lower vibrations. Feeling the high-frequency emotions and vibrations connects you to original source. When in this high vibration, it does not matter what you are thinking. You may just be present and happy, and abundance will flow to you. When you see high-vibration people, you will think, "Wow, everything good happens to them," or, "They are so lucky." It is not luck. It is the Laws of Attraction. We all know people who have the opposite happen to them. It seems they are always having "bad" things happen to them. They may say things like, "I am so unlucky, I always break things. Bad things always happen to me," and sure enough, event after event comes their way to make those beliefs true for them. These people seem to have the worst luck ever. They are walking accidents. Other beliefs like, "Whenever things start to go well something bad happens," or "Bad things happen in threes," will also come true if you believe them. The Laws of Attraction are behind it, whether you like it or not. "Ask, and it will be given to you; seek, and you will find; knock, and it will be opened to you. For everyone who asks receives, and the one who seeks finds, and to the one who knocks it will be opened." (Matthew 7:7–8 World English Bible). The Laws of Attraction can be found at the core of all spiritual teachings.

Universal Consciousness

All things you see around you had to be imagined first. From the one mind, the universe was created. We are always connected to the one mind, and with practice can learn to use that creative energy. Nobel Prize winner in Physics Max Plank said, "I can tell you as a result of my research about atoms this much: There is no matter as such! All matter originates and exists only by virtue of a force which brings the particles of an atom to vibration and holds this most minute solar system of the atom together …. We must assume behind this force the existence of a conscious and intelligent Mind. This Mind is the matrix of all matter."

Throughout the book, I will use different words for source energy: God, universal consciousness, love, spirit, quantum field, and Tao. There was a time when I refused to read or listen to anything with the word "God" in it. From childhood, I had been conditioned to believe that God was an old man lording over human beings from heaven, punishing those who are bad, then forgiving them when they asked for forgiveness. Throughout my spiritual journey, that has changed. I now see God as the universal consciousness, the oneness that we all return to and come from, the infinite force that creates life. You can use whichever word you prefer on your spiritual journey.

Self-Care and Self-Management

Self-care is vital to thrive in life. If we are giving to others from a state of lack, all we will get is more lack and a lot of resentment. We want to fill ourselves up first so we can give from abundance. When our needs are met, only then can we truly meet others' needs. Too often we spend all our time taking care of others because we are looking for love, approval, or appreciation. When our cup is full, we are able to give without needing this in return. Love, approval, and appreciation just become icing on the cake. Self-care and time-management go hand in hand. Whenever I mention self-care, I usually hear, "I do not have enough time for that." Mindset training is self-care. To me, it is the most important form of self-care. Things like massages, manicures, and other spa type treatments may feel like they are more important, but they are not. Those give much more temporary shifts in vibration. Mindset training, when done regularly, can give long-lasting shifts in vibration and allow you to stay in balance during times of stress.

Originally, this section was going to be called "Self-Care and Time-Management." Everyone has the same amount of time in a day, so the term time-management does not make any sense. We cannot manage time. We cannot slow it down or speed it up, nor can we stop it or put it into blocks. We can, however, manage ourselves and how we use our time. We can learn tools to make ourselves more efficient. One of those tools is delegation. In the book *The Big Leap,* Gay Hendricks teaches that we all have a zone of genius, tasks that only we can do, things that we are really good at and have a passion for. In order to make time for self-care, we want to delegate those things that are not in this category. When I first learned about this technique, it was hard for me to implement. To say that I was obsessive-compulsive would be an understatement. I felt I did things best, and because of this, I needed to do all the things. For instance, loading the dishwasher. My husband obviously never played the Nintendo game *Tetris* because he has no skills at getting a bunch of dishes to fit into the small dishwasher space. There is no order to his dishwasher loading. Everything just goes all over the place with so much space leftover. So of course, I had to unload and reload the dishwasher.

It can be difficult to give up control. The first part of the process is to recognize your need for it. Once you have awareness of it, you can then start telling yourself there is no right or wrong way to do things. My way may seem best to me, but other people may feel the same way about how they do it. Allowing people to do things the way they want is a great way to tame the ego, which we will discuss more in later sections. Common things to delegate either to other family members or to hired help are house cleaning, laundry, cooking, dishes, and yard maintenance. If you run a business, hiring an assistant to help with tasks like answering emails, placing orders, answering phone calls, shipping, data input, etc., will free up your time. *The 4-Hour Work Week* by Tim Ferriss is a great book on how to optimize your work schedule to do less and achieve more. It is all about working smarter, not harder.

The other thing that got me stuck on delegation was money. At the time I learned about delegation, I did not have family members, besides my husband, that could take over tasks. During that time, he was quite busy. I also did not have much money. My money mindset needed some fine-tuning. I took the leap of faith and began delegating cleaning and business tasks. This allowed me to spend more time on money-generating activities only I could do. Had I not delegated tasks, I would not have been able to build my business. Today, delegation is second nature to me. If I do not want to do it, you can bet it is delegated. My zones of genius are being a mom, client calls, test analysis, recording videos, writing, and self-care. When you first start delegating, it is best to start small. Delegate a few of the tasks you are doing. This will free up some time for self-care. As you get practice delegating, do more of it.

The other way we can delegate in the work world is through technology. My business is all streamlined using online tools like Customer Management Systems, courses, auto emails, etc. It took some time to set up, but now that it is all in place, I do not have to do much work outside of my zone of genius. People always think I must be so busy because I run my business, am a mom, write, and have a lot of time for self-care, but in reality, I feel I have lots of time because I delegate and streamline.

Exercise #2: Delegate: Make a list of the tasks only you can do and those you can delegate. Brainstorm how and to whom you will delegate the tasks.

Often, we feel that people are taking advantage of us, that we are doing everything and not getting help. In truth, we are allowing it. The following exercise can help you get clear on where you need to say "no" and set boundaries.

Exercise #3: Setting Boundaries: What are you allowing to happen in your life that drains you? Where do you need to set up healthy boundaries in your life? How will you change this pattern by setting healthy boundaries where they are needed? Where do you know it's time for you to say "no"?

Self-care is a priority for me. I include it in my zone of genius, as no one else can do my self-care for me. It is a must, and it is why I am able to handle stress well and stay in a peaceful state of mind, considering everything I manage. It is also a big part of staying healthy. Self-care comes in all sorts of shapes and sizes. For me, mindset is at the top. I do it daily and have for years. In the beginning, when I first started learning about mindset training, I spent every free moment on it, to an average of three to five hours a day.

My current mindset routine is what I have all my clients do. It includes daily meditation and listening to or reading mindset books. For me, an hour is minimum, and I most often listen to mindset books for two or more hours a day. Listening to mindset books is how I reprogram my brain from old thought patterns of lack, stress, anger, and anxiety to new ones of peace, love, and joy. These books bring repetition of concepts which, in time, will make its way into the subconscious and rewrite old limiting beliefs and thought patterns. Even after years of practice, I find if I go too many days without, I start reverting back.

This is because most people in the world are always making excuses, complaining, and blaming. Constantly listening to that brings the old patterns right back. I listen to mindset books while Kaiden sleeps and while I am driving in the car. Sometimes I listen to them on walks when I am alone, while juicing (when that is not being delegated), when cleaning (again, that is usually delegated but sometimes things happen, and I end up doing it), and at times I have my earphones in listening when Kaiden is playing. Usually, that only happens when I need an extra mindset kick due to triggers. Mindset books include any books on self-growth and self-development. There are many references to my favorites throughout this book.

The next most important part of my self-care is riding. I have been riding horses since I was twelve years old. Being at the barn with my horses and riding is at the top of my list of passions. There is nothing like the feeling of galloping through the woods on my horse. Going to the barn is rejuvenating. It also gives me a great energy and endorphin boost.

Other forms of self-care for me are hiking with my dogs, spending time with friends and family, massages, and at the bottom of the list, would be showers. It is nice to feel clean, but when it comes to managing self-care, it often gets shoved back. Riding is just way more fun, and who needs to be clean when you are just going to come home smelling like horse anyway?

Everyone's self-care is going to look different, though it is important to put mindset training at the top of your list. This includes making time for meditation and listening to or reading books. After that, get your passions in. Then get in the relaxation time. Some people find shopping to be therapeutic. Other ideas are sports, crafts, painting, long drives, pedicures, hair appointments, watching TV, doing nothing, salt caves, and cooking.

Another part of self-care is rest days. Some days, we just need to do nothing. Some days, the body feels like lazing around. I honor those days, even if I have a full schedule, I will move things around to respect my body. It is good to have one rest day a week where activity is kept to a lower degree. Often when the weather is bad, the body will want a rest day. On rest days, it is best to stick to your meditation and mindset schedule if you are in the first thirty days of creating a new habit. After that, you can use your mini meditation from "Part Three: Spirit" to bring yourself to presence. There definitely are days when I do not listen to mindset books, but those are few and far between. Since there is so much "negativity" in the world, I like to keep that going, as it helps to keep me centered.

Exercise #4: Get Clear on Your Self-Care: Take some time now to make a list of your self-care choices.

The next tool needed for self-management is scheduling. If it is not in your schedule, it is not going to get done. An agenda, day planner, calendar, or an app on your phone will work. Every Sunday, take time to schedule your mindset training into your calendar. After that, schedule in anything pertaining to work or family. Then put in times for your passions, and schedule in time for self-care.

I will use my typical day as an example. I delegate cleaning, which includes vacuuming, mopping, dusting, and bathrooms. I delegate juicing and baking. I delegate all yard work, house repair, snow shoveling, gardening, and dog poop cleaning. I do my own cooking and laundry. I try to ride a few times a week, though this can be more or less often depending on how much test analysis I have coming in and what the weather is like for riding. On my way home from riding, I do my shopping and errands. I schedule those into the calendar, also, so I do not spend time trying to remember what needs to be done. I like to get a massage or osteopath treatment once every second or third week, more often if I am very active and my muscles need more support.

	Monday	Tuesday	Wednesday	Thursday	Friday	Saturday	Sunday
8:00	Breakfast/ Walk/ Stretch	Breakfast/ Walk/ Stretch	Breakfast/ Walk/ Stretch	Breakfast/ Walk/ Stretch	Breakfast/ Walk/ Stretch	Breakfast/ Walk/ Stretch	Breakfast
9:00	Riding	Work	Riding	Family	Riding	Family	Family
10:00	Riding	Work	Riding	Family	Riding	Work	Family

11:00	Groceries	Work	Riding	Family	Groceries	Family	Family
12:00	Lunch	Lunch	Lunch	Lunch	Lunch	Lunch	Lunch
1:00	Family	Family	Family	Family	Family	Mindset	Family
2:00	Mindset	Mindset	Mindset	Mindset	Mindset	Mindset	Mindset
3:00	Family	Work	Work	Work	Work	Work	Family
4:00	Family	Work	Work	Work	Work	Family	Family
5:00	Dinner	Dinner	Dinner	Dinner	Dinner	Dinner	Dinner
6:00	Work	Work	Work	Work	Work	Work	Family
7:00	Work	Work	Work	Work	Work	Work	Family
8:00	Bedtime Routine	Bedtime Routine	Bedtime Routine	Bedtime Routine	Bedtime Routine	Bedtime Routine	Bedtime Routine
9:00	Watch Show	Watch Show	Watch Show	Watch Show	Watch Show	Watch Show	Watch Show
10:00	Write	Write	Write	Write	Write	Write	Write
11:00	Read	Read	Read	Read	Read	Read	Read
12:00	Bed	Bed	Bed	Bed	Bed	Bed	Bed

Scheduling is something we want to do to increase motivation to get things done and prevent forgetting. I use the calendar app in my phone and change the color from blue to black when I have done something on the list. That is a reward for my brain. My brain loves checklists. We do not want scheduling and self-care to become stressful. Scheduling every minute of the day to the point of OCD is not healthy. If you find yourself scheduling every minute of your day, make sure to add in "do nothing" times. With practice, including self-care into your life will become a habit. In my sample schedule where it says "work," it would have a list of things that need to be done. I sit down and get started on one at a time, checking each off as I go. If I do not get it done, it moves to the next work block. Under family, I may put the activity we are doing or just leave it as unscheduled time. We usually sit down and have all meals together as a family. Note that I do watch TV and write before bed. I do not have any trouble falling asleep or staying asleep. If insomnia is an issue, it is best to schedule this time away from blue light emitting technology.

Another tool that really aids in self-management is segmenting your day and your tasks, then taking a few minutes before each new segment to visualize it going smoothly. This activates the Laws of Attraction and helps bring about your intention. For example, when you step into your car, take a second to visualize your drive. See yourself getting green lights, responding calmly to other drivers, and arriving safely. If you are going shopping, take a second to see yourself getting a good parking spot, not standing in any lines, and easily finding what you need. In all visualizations, see yourself having fun and being relaxed, and see each task flowing to the next with ease. The same goes with work and home life. The visualization only needs ten to twenty seconds.

Before creating your schedule, you want to identify time wasters. A common time waster is the time we spend on unproductive thoughts. These can affect us in two ways. The first is that we become so consumed with our thoughts that they keep us from taking action. These can be thoughts about things that worry us, over-analysis of tasks, or obsessive thoughts around an argument or other trouble in life. The other way these thoughts waste time is when we do get into action, they prevent us from focusing on a task. This will make the task take a lot longer than it should. This is often labelled as ADD. In truth, concentration takes a lot of practice. The meditations in "Part Three: Spirit" will assist in this aspect of mindset training. You want to become aware of the thoughts that are distracting you and gently redirect yourself back to the task at hand.

The key to successful scheduling and self-management is mastering the dichotomy of "I have things on my list to do, but there is nothing I have to do." There really is nothing that has to be done besides eating, drinking, and breathing. We feel we have to go to work, clean the house, take care of the kids, but in reality, that could be put off until another time, or someone else could do it. We could sit and let the time pass and just be the observer, and that is totally okay. Eckhart Tolle did it. He just sat on a park bench for a long time. Getting to this point in my life has taken a lot of spiritual development. I see the grand scheme of the universe and how trivial daily tasks are. Every once in a while, I hear the thought come from my subconscious, "You have so much to do today."

I kindly remind it that there really is only the present moment. It will get done in its own time. The more I stay present, the more things get done, yet it seems I have less to do and more time to be.

"Einstein time" is the term used when time seems to stop, speed up, or slow down. The first time I experienced it was when I was meeting Eric and his mom at a restaurant at 5:00 p.m. I had a lot to do that day, and by Eric's standards, I was going to be late. I had a firm belief I would make it on time. It usually takes twenty to thirty minutes to get to the restaurant from my house. I texted him when I left the driveway and headed on my way. He told me I would be late because it was rush hour. Somehow, I got to the restaurant at 5:02 p.m. He was not there. When I looked at the time my text was sent, I had left at 4:50 p.m. I did not drive fast to get there, either. I just relaxed and listened to a mindset book on the way with the belief I would make it on time. When he walked into the restaurant, Eric was shocked to find me sitting at a table. I have since had multiple occasions where this has happened. I have the belief I will be on time. Perhaps my belief opens up the traffic to allow me to cruise there unimpeded. All I know is it is an incredible feeling. I often get in this zone when I am doing test analysis. I get so focused on the present moment that time seems to slow down, and I can get so much done in very little time. What would often take three hours is done in thirty-five minutes. The key is presence. When I sit down to work, I allow any distracting thoughts to pass through me. This skill has developed from years of meditation practice becoming the observer. The more you shift into the observer state, the easier life will flow.

Technology is a huge time waster and turning it off will add extra time to your day. How much TV do you watch? How long do you spend on social media? How often do you check your email? It is best to take social media off your phone. I only have my Kindle reader and Audible on my phone. If I need to look at my phone to serve my phone addiction, it will be to read or listen to a mindset book. Phone addiction is real. We get addicted to the scrolling eye movement. Notifications give us a boost in dopamine as do "likes" on posts. Turning off your phone may be one of the harder habits to break, but it is well worth it. Schedule in time to check those apps. Schedule how much TV you want to watch. Schedule how much time you play games. If you truly feel it is a form of self-care, then allow yourself a little bit of time per day to spend on it. If it becomes a need, it is time to see that it is an addiction. Addiction to technology may seem like a less harmful one than alcohol or drugs, but it is an addiction nonetheless and other more important things in life are passing you by. That time could be spent writing the book you always wanted to write, taking a course, spending time with family, or getting a better career. No one ever said on their death bed, "I wish I would have spent more time on my phone."

For people suffering from chronic illness, researching is not only a time waster, but it can also become an addiction. I know, as I was there once. Focusing on symptoms can get to a point of obsessive-compulsive behavior. Spending time in Facebook groups or other forums, getting stuck in victim mentality, is not only a time waster, it is damaging to our health. On my own journey, trial and error caused me harm. Get help, get proper testing to see what your body needs, and shift focus to healing. We get what we focus on, and if you are looking for illness or constantly reading about it, the odds are you are going to manifest it. When I first started working as a health coach, I had issues with manifesting clients symptoms. The same thing would happen when I would take courses. What I was focused on, I would start to see in my body. Luckily, the symptoms would not be long-term, but it was amazing to see. If I had a client who suffered from rashes, I would develop a rash. If clients would talk about yeast infections, I would get one. It took a lot of mindset training and separating my energy to get to a point where that stopped happening. If you are in Facebook groups reading about other people's symptoms and looking for diagnoses, then that is what you are focused on and will manifest.

Exercise #5: Identify Time Wasters: In order to make a schedule, you will want to first see what yours looks like now. Take a day or a week to monitor the time you spend on each task throughout the day. Go through the list above again, identify your time wasters, and write them in your calendar. If you spend fifteen minutes thinking, write it down. If you spend forty minutes on your phone on social media, write it down. This exercise will reveal where you tend to waste time. Once you know what your time wasters are, when you do them, and how long you spend on them, you can schedule in productive tasks and redirect yourself when you find yourself going back to a time waster.

Exercise #6: Create a Schedule: Once you have seen your current schedule, identified your time wasters, decided on self-care, and started to delegate tasks, take time at the end of each week to make a schedule for the coming week. Include in it your self-care, family time, and work. Use lists to get tasks out of your head so you are not wasting time thinking about them. Break tasks down into little steps that are easier to accomplish.

The Stages of Consciousness

I was first introduced to the stages of consciousness through Michael Beckwith's teachings and have heard it echoed from many other spiritual teachers along my spiritual journey. The stages of consciousness are not linear; people go back and forth between them, and in some areas of their lives may stay in one more than another. The more mindset training and spiritual growth that has been done; the more people stay in the higher stages. You can believe in your ability to influence your surroundings and remain in a state of allowance, especially toward the things you cannot change. There is no right or wrong in the stages of consciousness. It is not better to be in one stage or the other. Most people are here to just experience without being conscious. That is their journey.

Stage One is victim: The world happens to me. All power is given away to the event, and all happiness is looked for externally. People blame their pasts for where they are at now in life. The past becomes their excuses. Making excuses, complaining, and blaming are where their energy is focused. Excuses are victim stories and all the reasons why they have not been able to progress in life. When you make excuses, you are not taking responsibility. You are trying to blame an outside circumstance. Most of the population is at this stage. This is an outer-directed person.

Stage Two is manifestation. Taking responsibility moves a person from victim mentality into phase two consciousness. This is where one learns that through the power of thoughts and the Laws of Attraction, one can create one's own life. The way you respond to events creates the outcome, and you always have a choice in how you respond. Stage two is the beginning of inner direction, though much of the focus is often still on creating things to make you happy. Here the person uses their past to fuel them to higher levels. Their past is a lesson, a blessing. One learns that for manifestation to happen, focus needs to be on feeling happy with what is present now and on finding gratitude and love no matter the events. This realization shifts the person to stage three.

Stage Three is allowance. Whatever comes is accepted as exactly how it should be. The universe is perfect. Trust and faith in the universe and oneself define this stage.

Stage Four is oneness. It means being totally one with the universal consciousness. The people who reach this stage are few and include great teachers like Jesus, Buddha, Mother Theresa, Saint Francis of Assisi, and Krishna.

Peace and happiness are the goals of spiritual growth. Most people in stage one consciousness are not happy unless their environment is providing it for them. I also believe that before coming here, we make an agreement with other beings to help each other experience, learn, and grow. Some people who seem to be stuck in phase one consciousness and cause stress in our lives are divine beings here to teach us. They may do some terrible acts. Through those acts, we learn forgiveness and compassion. The suffering is needed to bring us to the next stage of consciousness. I believe this happens on a world scale, also. Certain beings in history commit terrible acts that lead to global awakening.

Exercise #7: Awareness Check: Check in on where you believe you are in the stages of consciousness. Remember, there is no right or wrong. We are aiming for awareness. Shed some light on where you are so you can set a course for where you want to be. Perhaps in some areas of your life, you are in stage one most of the time; in others, you are in stage two or three. As you move farther into the book, there will be more exercises to help move out of stage one consciousness.

The Stages of Enlightenment

The stages of enlightenment are different than the stages of consciousness and are how one finds spiritual growth and revelation through their experiences. In hindsight, I truly believe that the illnesses I went through on my own healing journey were to promote spiritual growth. Had I not gotten ill, I would most likely be an exhausted massage therapist with a violent temper and severe emotional issues, always living paycheck to paycheck with no sense of inner joy or purpose. On my journey, I was introduced to the Laws of Attraction and mindset training, both of which have changed not only my health but every aspect of my life. They have allowed me to create happy relationships and a successful business, find my purpose, and face my fears of getting pregnant. Had I not gotten sick, none of these would have happened. Overcoming my illness has given me knowledge and tools to help others overcome their illness. Had I not gone through that suffering, I would not have been able to be of service to others. It is always amazing to get messages from total strangers telling me how much I have helped them on their journeys through my videos and writings.

I believe there are three stages of enlightenment. Many people do not experience any enlightenment or awakenings in their lifetime. These people go through life unconscious, in stage one consciousness, then they die and reincarnate without ever having learned the power of their thoughts.

1. The first stage of enlightenment is awakening and becoming conscious of how suffering through an event has caused self-growth. This happens after a person has made it through to the other side and can look back with the realization that the event had a purpose. I suffered for many years with illness. After I was

through the suffering, I could look back and say it was perfect. It was exactly what I needed to grow. After reaching this stage of enlightenment where one realizes the power of one's thoughts and that there is something to be learned through all suffering, a person can move to the second stage.

2. The second stage of enlightenment is when a person sees every event as it is happening as a way to grow. These people look for the silver lining and the lesson while they are suffering. Kaiden's birth was very hard on my body. For months afterward, I could barely walk. My pelvic floor suffered a significant prolapse. My physiotherapist told me not to do anything that caused symptoms. Walking caused symptoms, so I spent most of the first five months after giving birth on a chair in my living room. I could have been depressed and upset. Instead, I focused on gratitude for having a beautiful baby boy. I found the silver lining and took the time to dive into genetics and how they affected detoxification and neurotransmitter expression. I turned something that could have been stressful and depressing into an enlightening experience.

3. The third stage of enlightenment is getting out ahead. This getting out ahead comes from a place of peace, not from a place of constant anxiety and planning. It is facing fears before they happen, learning mental tools to face any event, staying peaceful, and seeing where conflict may occur in the future, and defusing conflict before it starts. The third stage prevents suffering or reduces the time of suffering. Learning and spiritual growth become a daily practice.

I believe that until you learn a lesson, it will keep repeating in your life. We see this often in relationships, where the person will repeat the same abusive relationship. They break free of one but do not do the work on self-confidence and self-love, so they attract the exact same qualities in their next partner.

To move up these stages of enlightenment, energy needs to be moved out of the physical journey. Our physical journey includes our work, relationships, and finances. Instead, we put that energy into our spiritual journey. This involves turning inward through meditation and listening to or reading spiritual books, attending seminars, taking courses, etc. The amazing thing is that our spiritual growth will in turn bring growth to our physical journeys.

When Kaiden was born, I developed intense anxiety around him dying. My spiritual focus shifted to changing my beliefs around death and working through these fears. Over the past few years, I had developed trust that the answer I was looking for would come to me if I asked. Every step of the way has seemed to always fall into place, and I trust that now.

Since Kaiden was young, travelling to spiritual teachers was not going to happen, so I turned to audiobooks. I immersed myself in Byron Katie, Wayne Dyer, and Caroline Myss, meditating on the questions I had. Through meditation, I discovered the answers I was seeking. I got out ahead of these fears to be prepared for anything that could come my way. If Kaiden was to die, I know I would be okay in time. Of course, nothing we do can prevent the pain of losing a loved one, but we can develop tools to help us not be destroyed by it. Though I have a fear of him dying, I no longer feel anxiety. I know this fear is a normal survival mechanism and am grateful for it. It helps me keep him safe. Though the thought may come, I do not entertain it by visualizing him dying. I recognize the fear, show my gratitude for it, and redirect myself. Along this journey, I also realized that I was trying to find something, anything, to keep me from having to feel the pain of loss. A truth I found was that we come here to experience all emotions. I truly believe we chose to be here, with certain people, to experience certain things, to learn and grow. When I think that my higher self is okay with whatever happens in this life, it brings me peace.

Exercise #8: Awareness Check: Check in to see where you are in the stages of enlightenment. Are you mostly in stage one and seeing only the good in a situation after you are through it? Or are you in stage two and starting to look for lessons and silver linings while you are going through an event? Or perhaps you are starting to get out ahead and face your fears in stage three.

Empowering Language

The language we use to talk to others and ourselves is very important when activating the Laws of Attraction. Our language is also vital to how our bodies feel. Most people are not aware of the language they use or the power it has. Our thoughts are mostly words. Even if an image comes across our minds, the little voice in our head will quickly name it. Resting our awareness on something without naming it requires practice. We want to learn to become aware of the language we are using and choose language that helps shift us into a high vibration. Language that empowers us and makes our bodies feel good. Shifting to empowering language is meant to be fun. You have been speaking to yourself in the manner that you do for your entire life. Most of the world speaks with a lot of negativity. Be gentle with yourself when shifting your language, as it will take time and practice to create a new inner voice.

The first step in shifting from language that weakens you to language that empowers you is to be aware of the words "I am." God said, "I am that I am." (Exodus 3:14 KJV) The words "I am," are incredibly powerful. "I am," is a command to your higher self. It defines who you are and what you can do. Any words that follow "I am," should be constructive and of high vibration. Saying "I am sick," sends a powerful message to the subconscious. Instead, say, "Today I feel sick," if you must describe how you are feeling. You can also say, "My body feels sick." This way you are not labeling yourself. You are just describing what your body feels. It is also a great step in dissociation from the body. The more we dissociate from the body, the more suffering becomes optional. Dissociation from the body will help you become the observer.

Take a second to say each, right now: "I am sick," versus "I feel sick," versus "My body feels sick." There is a big difference. Try "I am stupid," versus "I feel stupid," versus "My actions were stupid." Again, there is a big difference. When you notice you are diminishing yourself with low-vibration words after the words "I am," take a few seconds to make the shift. Do this by choosing a new phrase and repeating it a few times out loud (or in your head if people are around). For example, if you said, "I am so dumb. Why do I always do stupid things?" Affirm a few times, "I am a genius; I choose to learn from my past and will make better choices in the future."

I have practiced this a lot over the years, and I notice when other people do it. It is really clear where our low self-confidence comes from. Most people are always putting themselves down. We will learn more in subsequent sections about how this inner critic that often berates us comes from childhood, when we were often scolded for making mistakes. The great thing is that you do not have to go back into the past and undo every event that caused trauma. To create a new belief and shift your inner critic into an inner coach just takes repetition. For now, practice noticing what you say after the words "I am," and repeat a higher-vibration choice. If another person says something negative after the words "I am," give them a compliment or try to raise them up. If they are not ready to accept that, simply repeat a higher choice of words in your own mind. This way you are cancelling it out and putting what you do want to hear into your subconscious.

Step two in shifting to empowering language is to be aware of lower-vibration words. Personally, if I do something stupid, I choose to say, "I am a genius." I do not say it sarcastically, either. Instead, I bring to mind times when I have been a genius, in order to shift my vibration. I use the times I have been really smart to counterbalance the event that just occurred that caused me to feel stupid. Another example would be to choose a playful word like "silly." Lower-vibration words can be fun to shift. Be creative. The premise is that if I say, "Do not think about a yellow horse," you will see a picture of a yellow horse in your mind. Words are powerful, and if you practice speaking only what you want to manifest, it can change your life.

You do not have to obsess over it or get upset when you choose lower-vibration words. Though words are powerful, our feelings are even more so. If you are getting upset about your language, it will not matter what you are saying, as the feeling of anger will be your vibration. Simply become aware of the language you are using. When you are making your own affirmations, be sure to use empowering words like "healthy," "powerful," "abundant," "joyful," and "creative." Avoid words like "sick," "debt," and "illness." "I am happy I am financially free," is more powerful than "I am happy I am out of debt." "I am grateful I am healthy and vibrant," is more powerful than "I am grateful I am no longer sick." Ideally, remove those words from your vocabulary. It is easy to do in affirmations, as you consciously create them. We will work on creating affirmations in another section. Our inner dialogue and the way we speak takes much more practice. The way we talk to others and ourselves has been programmed from childhood, so expect it to take time to change.

Examples of empowering words are: smart, passionate, strong, capable, successful, calm, kind, determined, adventurous, talented, respected, loved, beautiful, charming, motivated, brave, interesting, free, spirited, joyful, graceful, energetic, confident, assertive, unique, abundant, ambitious, authentic, blessed, creative, powerful, dedicated, divine, driven, excited, fierce, genius, insightful, purposeful, radiant, sensual, and stunning.

Confusing words would be a word like "fearless." You would think that would be an empowering word, but because the word "fear" is in it, the subconscious will focus on that. Other examples of confusing words are "unbreakable" and "unstoppable." The mind sees "break" and "stop."

One of my least favorite words is "bad." Telling someone they are "bad" really affects the subconscious. Everyone wants to be good. Feeling like a bad person and the fear of being a bad person stops people in their tracks and affects self-worth. It is a word I do not use in my house. Even if the dog does something like pee in my bed, I do not say it is a bad dog. I will use the word "naughty," if needed, as it gives a more playful sense. Everyone makes mistakes. It does not mean they are a bad person. It is vital to see past behaviors to the person's inner being.

Examples of disempowering words are: bad, hard, fail, evil, stupid, sick, disease, fat, and ugly. Disempowering words also include any swear words.

If you find yourself feeling any of the disempowering words, bring to mind its opposite. For example, if you are feeling tired, remember a time you felt energetic. If you are feeling sick, remember a time you felt healthy. If you are feeling scared, remember a time you felt brave. Acknowledge and respect how you feel. "Today, I feel tired. I choose to *find* energy." This way is more believable for many people who feel just stating what they want is lying to themselves. Use the transitional word "find" and with practice, graduate to "Today I feel tired. I choose *to be* energetic." In time, you can affirm "I am energetic," and believe it.

Step three in shifting to empowering language is to recognize when you are complaining. Whenever you complain, you will attract more to complain about. If you are around others who are complaining, you do not help them by being a sounding board for their complaints. Complaining will block receiving. Recognize complaining and choose to refocus with more empowering language. When you are complaining, you are most likely using lower-vibration language and judging others. Instead, focus on people's strengths. When you focus on what you love in a person, you will get more of that quality. This is why in our morning meditation (see "Part Three: Spirit"), we focus on appreciation of ourselves and another person. Shifting into appreciation and gratitude by choosing language of praise is a powerful tool in manifestation. When you feel yourself complaining about something, try to find something you are grateful for. For example, the day before writing this section, I was getting ready to go to sleep and noticed my dog had peed in my bed. Most people would have been very upset. Instead, I focused on being grateful that I had just recently purchased a new set of sheets and a new mattress protector, both of which were washed and ready to go. I also focused on having clean sheets, as I love the feeling of fresh sheets. I was thankful to whichever one of my three dogs told me it was a good time to enjoy fresh sheets. I went to bed with feelings of gratitude instead of anger and annoyance.

When you stop complaining, the first thing you will notice is how much everyone else complains. They complain about the weather, work, spouses, friends, and money. Watch that you do not start complaining about how much other people complain. The truth is you can change any situation, but you are choosing not to because of some benefit, or it is too hard to make the change. You have a reference point for something that is better, but you do not want to take the risk or put the effort in to get it. It is much easier to stay in your comfort zone. Our bubble of ease. It may not be exactly what you want, but it is safe. It is safer than the unknown, which demands we face our fears and stretch ourselves. Say, for example, you do not like the weather where you live. You can always move somewhere else. You are not willing to take the risk and face the challenges of moving, so you stay stuck and complain. I had a client start working on mindset, and within six months, she had moved herself and her family across the country to a warmer climate. With the help of mindset training and by learning she could do whatever she put her mind to, she was able to manifest a better job for her husband. She faced huge fears moving away from her family. Now, she is living her dream life on the beach.

Instead of complaining about a person, tell them how you feel. If you do not like the situation you are in, you can always leave. If you do not want to face the fears, that is fine, too. Accept the situation.

Make sure you are not complaining to the wrong person. If you are having issues with your spouse, tell your spouse, not your friends. Your friends cannot change your spouse's behavior. No one can but your spouse, and if you do not face the fear of confrontation, then your spouse will never have the opportunity to change. In the "Building Healthy Relationships" section, we will go over tools to help you learn to communicate effectively without triggering the other person.

Exercise #9: Give Up Complaining: Where are you complaining in life? What are you not willing to risk in order to create your ideal life? What fears are keeping you stuck?

Step four in shifting to empowering language is to lose the word "need" from your vocabulary. Byron Katie said, "To think you need something you do not have is the definition of insanity." If you truly needed it, it would be here. When you say the word "need," you are putting yourself into a state of lack. You are focusing on what you do not have and telling the universe you do not have enough. Our feeling is our attraction point so you will get more lack. The key to attracting anything is to give up attachment to the outcome. If you find yourself often using the words "I need," recognize that and make a change to focusing on what you desire. The more you shift it, the more it will become habit. See what you want as already manifested. Live as though you already have it, be okay with not having it, and trust it will show up in the right time. It is one of the great dichotomies to master and the ultimate attraction point. Shifting to gratitude for what you do have will move you out of lack.

Step five in shifting to empowering language is to give up the words "I can't." With the proper training and time, you can do most anything you put your mind to. Saying, "I can't," gives your power away. Almost always you can do it, but you choose not to. Acknowledge that and use empowering language, such as, "I choose not to," instead of "I can't." Usually, "I can't," is followed by a line of excuses for why you can't. Instead say, "I choose." You can still say why you are choosing not to, but you are owning your power. If you think something is difficult, instead of putting power there, say, "This is a challenge. I choose to accept it. I am handling it with ease." The language you use all the time and what you say or hear will become your beliefs. Make sure those beliefs are ones that serve your highest good.

Step six in choosing empowering language is to stop trying. Try to bend down and pick up something off the floor. Do not actually do it. Just try. Keep trying. It is not fun to keep trying without results. When you say, "I will try," you are giving yourself the escape just in case you do not get it done. The end result will be you will have more things to try for and never get. Commit to the end result of doing. Believe you are going to do it, and then do it. When we learn to do affirmations, we always state it in the present tense as though what we want in the future has already manifested. "I am so grateful that I am driving my new blue Cadillac Escalade." We do not say, "I am so grateful I am trying to get my new Escalade." Recognize when you get stuck in the processes. Be aware of why you use the words "I will try to do my best," versus "I am going to have this done." The reason is fear of failure. You reject your own success now because you are afraid you might not get there. The easiest way to get rid of fear of failure is to recognize there is no such thing as failure. There is only learning. When Thomas Edison invented batteries, he had to try thousands of times before he got it right. When asked how it felt to have failed that many times, he said, "I did not fail; I now know a thousand ways not to make a battery." As long as you keep moving toward your goal, you have never failed. The same goes for "I will do that." When? Be specific. "I hope I can get it done tomorrow." You may always be hoping. Hoping is a great first step from disbelief, but do not get stuck in hoping. Hoping still leaves some room for doubt. Commit and be sure. I am. Channel your inner creative connection to source energy. Using empowering language will transfer the feeling and attraction point to you.

Step seven in shifting to empowering language is to lose the buts. They say anything after a "but" is crap. "You've done a really great job, but you forgot this." Anything before the "but" loses all value. Instead, use the word "and." "I love you, but you are a jerk," versus "I love you, and I am setting this boundary." The word "and" feels so much better.

Step eight in shifting to empowering language is to drop the labels. Whenever we judge others, we are finding fault. The ego is making us feel superior. Any judgment will be using disempowering labels. Judging others shows us areas within ourselves that need work. Learning to accept people for who they are and accept things for how they are, makes life much more peaceful. The ego kicks in and becomes defensive when we are triggered. Judging is saying we are right, and someone else is wrong. There is no right or wrong or good or bad. It is only a matter of perception and perspective. We often are projecting our beliefs of how things should be onto other people. We want to look at our own beliefs of what is right and wrong and see if they really are our own. Where did they come from? Do they serve us? People should not have to behave a certain way to make you happy. Instead, be honest about how things make you feel. "When you do _____, I feel _____." Instead of, "You make me feel ____." Remember you are choosing the response.

Before I learned this, whenever I saw a pretty girl, I would try to knock her down. This would make me feel better about myself. Now when I see someone, I find a compliment. I focus on the good. If someone else is judging, then I change the subject. Do not judge the person judging. I am not perfect at this all the time. It is a work in progress, and I welcome any aid in becoming aware of when I shift back to judging. Everyone has insecurities. Get the tools in place so we can start to see the good in ourselves and others. When you focus on the good in others, you will start to focus on the good in yourself. Giving a compliment instead of a judgment is choosing empowering language instead of disempowering. The other type of judgment we use is labels. These are especially detrimental to children. The labels we put on children end up being their limiting beliefs as adults. Calling a child a "sucky baby" or a "momma's boy" impacts the subconscious. The same happens when calling a child stubborn, bossy, or hyperactive. As a child, I had a voice. I was smart, I had an opinion, and I wanted to be heard. Then adults squashed it out of me, calling me bossy and telling me to be seen and not heard. Over and over, they put labels on me. Those labels stuck, and I had to undo them and create empowering beliefs. I am not bossy; I have leadership skills. It took thousands of hours and tens of thousands of dollars to reprogram my beliefs and to find my voice and confidence again. I now know that I do have leadership skills. I run a successful corporation while being a mom, writing, running a house, and practicing self-care. Had I not worked through the limiting beliefs I had about myself, none of these achievements would ever have been possible. This is why it is so important to watch the labels we put on others. We all remember Thumper on the movie *Bambi* saying, "If you can't say something nice, do not say nothing at all." It is true. Choose kindness and compassion. Choose to motivate and inspire. Choose to lift someone up instead of putting them down.

By not using labels, we also honor our feelings as things that will pass. Our feelings are not who we are. Children go through normal developmental periods. They bite, throw tantrums, can be stubborn, can be shy, and can be scared. It does not mean they will be like that forever. The same happens to adults. When we label them, we definitely increase the chances that they will become the label. Not labeling shows compassion and understanding. If someone is having a meltdown, child or adult alike, and is losing their temper, instead of calling them grouchy or an angry person, we just recognize they are having a bad day and need work on a skill in that area. When you see everyone as a divine spiritual being, all judgments, and labels dissolve.

I have put firm boundaries in place around language used toward Kaiden by adults in his life. We do not label him. I often hear in response, "Well, if he does not get used to it now, how will he cope in life?" I recognize that the world can be mean at times, and I understand he will come in contact with people who will call him names. I will give him skills to be confident in himself and believe other people's opinions of him are not a reflection of who he is. However, there is no reason for any child to be bullied by an adult who knows better and has a fully functioning frontal lobe. He will see how I stand up for him and myself and how I set boundaries as to what I feel is healthy for us. What we model, our children learn. The adults who care for him should be shields from wounds, not the cause of them.

When you begin to change your language from disempowering to empowering, you will start to notice other people's language. Whenever we learn something, we will first see how other people are lacking in those skills. This goes for anything. It is much easier to be aware of what other people are doing instead of what we are doing. It is another way the ego props itself up: "I am right, you are wrong. I am conscious, and you are not." When you hear someone else speaking with disempowering language, it is best not to coach them. This is your journey; lead by example. See how changing your language affects how you feel and how it changes your life. No one likes to be told what to do, especially family and friends. If they are interested, you can talk to them about the Laws of Attraction. Do not be surprised if you meet resistance. Often, as you learn these tools and become less reactive, the people closest to you will feel threatened and become triggered. It is the crab in the bucket phenomenon.

If you put a bunch of crabs in a bucket, you do not have to put a lid on because if one crab tries to escape, the others will pull it back down. This happens in our lives, also. When you start to make changes and grow spiritually, you will find the crabs around you will try to keep you from succeeding. They will mirror any doubts you may have about what you are doing and learning. It is part of the process. Focus on what feels right to you. Feel for those true beliefs and knowing. Go by what resonates with your being.

Protect Your Energy

As we begin our mindset journey, it is very important to limit time with energy drainers. Energy drainers are people in a chronic lower vibrational state. They are stuck in stage one consciousness and can be angry, judgmental, or verbally abusive. You know you are around an energy drainer when you are in a good mood, come into connection with them, and your energy just drains. Most of the time energy drainers are completely unconscious of their behavior. They are not purposely trying to drain your energy. They are just stuck in victim mentality. Many are addicted to this low frequency energy and feed off it, as it is the only thing they have. You may become tired and irritated yourself when you are around them. We all have these days once in a while. However, chronic energy drainers spend most of their time in this place. When you begin your mindset journey, they may put down your decision and discourage you in order to keep you at their level. When starting out on our mindset journeys, it is very easy to fall back into old thought patterns. It does not take much time around people in victim mentality for a person to shift back to that space.

Our goal with mindset training is to get to a place where other people's energy does not affect us; we are working to get to a place where we are living from abundance. When we get to this place, we become lighthouses for others, lifting people up without a drain on our own energy. Until that happens, it is best to limit your time spent with energy drainers, as they will easily bring you back to that level. It is important to find compassion for these people, as the odds are at some point in your life, you have been in the same place. We recognize and accept that they are not ready to change, but you are. To do so, you want to surround yourself with people who inspire, encourage, and motivate you. People who want you to succeed and be happy, and they may even try to assist you with ideas and resources. They may also introduce you to other people who think positive and are in a high-vibrational state most of the time. A great place to find people who are focused on self-growth and mindset is at your local Toastmasters. Toastmasters is a safe place people go to conquer their fear of public speaking. When I first started on my mindset journey, I did not think there were any like-minded people in my town. I joined Toastmasters, and to my delight, many people there were on the same journey of self-development.

Exercise #10: Identify Drainers and Motivators: Make a list of people you spend time with regularly. It can be friends, family, and coworkers. How do you feel around each person most of the time? Put a heart beside people that are inspiring and motivating. Put a check beside people who are neutral. These people may not be inspiring, but they do not drain your energy. Put an x beside people who drain your energy. You do not have to remove all your energy drainer friends from your life; just be conscious about how much time you spend with them until you get to a place where their energy does not bring you back to stage one consciousness.

Sometimes toxic people are our family members or coworkers, and we cannot avoid them. If that is the case, a tool to help offset their energy is to change the subject when they get into victim mode. Be clear about your venture into mindset work. Explain what you are working on and ask them to respect your choice. Learn to say "no," and set boundaries on the language used in your presence. I have people in my life who do not get along well together and have set the boundary to not have them come to my house at the same time because I do not want Kaiden to experience yelling, name-calling, etc. Personally, it does not have an effect on my energy, but it has taken work to get there. For a long time, it was very draining.

Often, when we begin to set boundaries with friends and family, energy drainers will try to guilt or manipulate you. They may tell you that you are being selfish. This will trigger our basic need for approval when self-confidence is low.

Exercise #11: Protect Your Energy: If you do need to spend time with energy drainers, use this visualization to help keep your energy. As often as you can remember or when you feel their energy getting to you, visualize a bubble or shield around you. You can also see your aura expanding. See any energy from these people as bouncing off your bubble of light. As you breathe in, continue to fill your bubble with peaceful blue or white light.

After taking my dogs for a walk in the baseball field by our hockey arena, I was putting Kaiden in the van when I heard a father yelling at his son. I looked and saw a man yelling at a boy who looked to be around five years old. They were far away, so I could not see it clearly. I got hit by a wave of anger, sadness, and pain. I could feel both of their emotions from across a parking lot. I started to cry and at the same time wanted to snap at Eric for not moving quicker. I was channeling both the child's and father's emotions. I felt so much empathy for the little boy being berated and shamed by his father. I was totally caught off guard and was not protecting my energy. This field is usually a very peaceful place. On the drive home, I had to cleanse my energy and find compassion for the father who obviously has had his own share of trauma in childhood to feel the need to yell and shame his child like that. I had to remind myself of my belief that both parent and child chose each other to teach each other and create experiences. Now when I go to the field, I do the above visualization and surround myself in a bubble of light, so I am not caught off guard again. Feeling another person's feelings and taking on their pain is a form of unhealthy empathy.

Building Confidence and Self-Love

Lack of self-confidence and self-love is detrimental to creating your ideal life and feeling peace and joy. Low self-confidence and self-love sound like:

"You are not good enough."

"You do not do things right."

"You always mess up."

"You do not deserve to be happy."

"You are weak."

"You are fat."

"You are ugly."

I purposely used the word "you" instead of "I." This is because we all have a voice in our heads that talks to us: our inner critic. For most people, they hear their inner voice judging them and judging others. This inner voice comes from how people talked to us when we were children. (See the "Conscious Parenting" section for more details on how it develops.) When we recognize that the voices we hear are not true, we can work to transform the critic into a coach. Confidence sounds like:

"I do not care what other people think of me or my actions."

"I follow my instincts."

"I am strong."

"I am beautiful."

"I can handle anything that comes my way."

"I am good."

Confidence is not being cocky. It is not being selfish. You can be unconcerned with the opinions of others and still speak with kindness and compassion. You can be confident in yourself and love who you are and still work on self-growth.

When someone says something to you that upsets you, it means part of you believes it to be true. It is something you need to work on to create more confidence in yourself around that belief. No one can truly hurt your feelings. It is not what someone says to you, it is what you say to yourself when the other person stops talking. If someone said to me that I am a terrible coach, it would not hurt me at all. I know deep down I am doing my absolute best to help all my clients. If I lacked confidence in myself, then the comment would hurt. Anytime you are triggered, it is your responsibility to dig deep and see why. It is a gift. What someone says is just another event. We get to choose how we respond to it. It is an opportunity for further personal growth. How other people treat you is their path, and how you respond is yours. The following are exercises I have found to be helpful in developing and increasing self-love and self-confidence.

Mirror Work

Mirror work is an exercise pioneered by Louise Hay that helps build confidence and self-love. It is easy to do yet is one of the things most people resist. Common resistance includes:

"I cannot look myself in the eyes."

"It feels too uncomfortable."

"I get angry, sad, nervous, etc. when I try to do it."

"I am afraid someone will walk in on me."

It is sad that we spend all day talking to ourselves, often berating ourselves, but we cannot look into the mirror and say some nice things to ourselves. Mirror work is just that, looking at yourself in the mirror and saying nice things about yourself. It is normal to feel all the aforementioned fears when starting this exercise. It is just a sad reality that society is this way. Ideally, kids should grow into adults who love and appreciate their bodies and their beings. Let us make having self-confidence and self-love the "new normal." It is never too late to start and always the right time to teach your kids or any other children in your life. Mirror works helps to turn your inner critic into your inner coach.

Exercise #12: Mirror Work: Stand in front of a mirror or hold your camera or handheld mirror so you can see yourself. Start by looking in the mirror into your own eyes and say, "(Your Name), you are beautiful.

(Your Name), I am proud of you. (Your Name), you are enough. (Your Name), I love you. Thank you, body, for carrying around my spirit." Do this once or twice a day or ideally every time you look into a mirror. If people are around, say it in your head. As you become more comfortable, you can increase the time spent in front of the mirror and go over any achievements you are proud of, acknowledging and thanking your body. It is best to always end with, "I love you." To create a new habit, try doing it for thirty days in a row.

Celebrate Success

One of the best ways to build confidence is to focus on and celebrate our successes in life. When you focus on what you want, you will get more of the same through the Laws of Attraction. When you know you have had success in the past, it will motivate you to take risks to create new successes.

Exercise #13: Celebrate Success: Write a list of twenty successes you have had in your life.

Exercise #14: Daily Success: Each day, celebrate five successes at the end of your day. These do not have to be life changing. It can be anything. Examples are: completing one page for your book, completing a task at work, completing your emails, eating healthy, avoiding temptations, going to bed at a reasonable hour, exercising, minimizing screen time, getting your mindset work done, cleaning a room or your house, and getting up on time.

Focus on Your Strengths

Most people have been programmed from childhood to not compliment themselves. It is seen as bragging, which is labelled as cocky, arrogant, and egotistical. Self-confidence is often squashed out of kids at a young age. The ego is responsible for this. Other people do not want you to feel good about yourself because it makes them feel smaller and jealous. So, they label and judge you. There is a difference between cockiness and self-love. There is a difference between arrogance and celebrating success. You are not responsible for what other people think of you. You can be sure of and proud of yourself while still being a compassionate being. You can also lead by example and inspire others to do the same. When someone compliments you, accept it and say, "thank you." Try to compliment others, and you will receive the same. The more you compliment others instead of judging them, it will help implant that response into your subconscious.

Exercise #15: Focus on Your Strengths: Get a blank piece of paper and write down everything you love about yourself. Use big letters and colorful pens or pencils. Ask your family and friends what they love about you and add it to the page. Read the page daily.

Find Your Inner Coach

This is a very powerful exercise I learned at *Train the Trainer* with Jack Canfield. From childhood, people are concerned about your well-being and do not always express it in a loving way. When we do something unsafe, instead of feeling that our parents' love is trying to protect us, we instead feel put down, judged, or punished because of how they express their concern. For example, as a child you break free from your parents and run across the road. When your parents get to you, in their anger, they tell you, "Why did you do that? Are you stupid? You could have gotten killed!" This will repeat thousands of times throughout most people's childhoods because most children do things that are dangerous, and they get reprimanded by their parents. Their criticism and voices are then inside you. When you do something you do not like, you berate yourself, just as the adults in your life berated you. Let's look at why they do this.

The first layer of emotion is anger, which is what they expressed when they found you doing something wrong or unsafe. Most people have heard this from their parents, and the cycle repeats itself. They only get to anger because they are still in stage one consciousness. The anger pattern is hardwired into their brains and takes work to change. The anger can also be seen as a punishment and in operant conditioning, punishment is believed to prevent future like behavior. They believe that punishment is the parenting model that works. The problem is, we are not animals. We have a subconscious, and the labels end up becoming not only our inner voice but the person we believe ourselves to be. Once you recognize that underneath the anger are the true feelings, you can bring out those emotions in yourself and have compassion toward how the adults responded when you were a child. The goal is to move deeper into the underlying emotions and learn to express them instead of the primitive feeling of anger.

The second deeper emotion is fear. The fear of loss. In the above example, instead of the adult saying, "You are so stupid. Why did you run across the road? You could have been killed," a better option would have been to say, "Please do not run across the road again. You could have been killed. I am so afraid of losing you."

The third deeper emotion is desire. "I desire to keep you safe. Please do not run across the road." Saying it this way feels even better.

The fourth deeper emotion is love. "I love you. Please stay close to me. I do not want to lose you."

Do you see the difference? Even though your parents and other adults in your life may have gotten angry with you, the truth is they were afraid to lose you. They wanted to keep you safe, and they love you so much. They were just stuck in a primitive emotion of anger, as they were conditioned by the way their parents spoke to them and were repeating the cycle. Get in touch with those deeper emotions and their true love for you in order to help heal those past hurts. Through this exercise, understand where your inner critic comes from, so you can find love for yourself. Learn to tap into those deeper emotions when talking to yourself and others. Doing this will further instill your own inner coach and help develop it in others.

Exercise #16: Move from Anger to Love: Make a list of all the things you say when you are judging yourself. Include all of the things you tell yourself you should do, but you do not do. Next, go through each criticism individually by passing it through the four emotions of anger, fear, desire, and love. Turn each one around. The criticism itself is anger. For example, using the criticism of, "You are so fat!" (Anger.) This will transform to, "I am afraid I will not lose weight and people will judge me." (Fear.) This will transform to, "I desire to be slim and loved." (Desire.) This will transform to, "I love my body; it deserves to be healthy. I deserve to be loved." (Love.)

When you find yourself being critical, tell the critic to stop, and then go through these steps to find the love behind it.

Create Your Ideal Life

It is so important when healing to shift focus from what we do not want (symptoms and illness) to what we do want. The first step in manifesting your ideal life is to decide what it is you want. Most people have never considered what it is they truly desire. We are molded from a young age by our parents and other adults to become something, ideally something great that makes a lot of money. Their egos take over and often shape our life paths. We suppress what we desire in order to make our parents happy, or we do the exact opposite to make them angry. Often, there are limiting beliefs that cause us to believe we do not deserve to be happy, successful, or wealthy. There are most likely limiting beliefs present that make us feel we do not have the ability to create our ideal lives, so we do not even bother thinking about it. After all, we would probably not succeed, anyway. We may have been taught to dream small to not to be disappointed. (See the "Limiting Beliefs" section to learn to recognize limiting beliefs and work through them.)

When you feel ready, even if you still have limiting beliefs present, work on visualizing your ideal life. Just knowing that you can create the life of your dreams and being aware that those limiting beliefs did not come from you is enough to move on to this step while you still work on creating empowering beliefs through repetition. Always remind yourself that everything you see in the world today first started out as a thought. If other people have this ability to create things from thought, so do you.

Exercise #17: Create Your Ideal Life: Get three pieces of paper. At the top of one, write "Financial and Career." At the top of the second one, write "Health and Body." At the top of the third one, write "Relationships and Personal." For this exercise, refer to the "Create Your Ideal Life Meditation" in "Part Three: Spirit" to assist in this process if needed. You can also just write down what you desire in these areas. When doing this exercise, let go of any limiting beliefs. Dream big. You can always refine it later, and it is normal for it to change over time. Be as detailed as possible.

Financial and Career: What is your ideal annual income and monthly income? How much money do you have in savings? What is your total net worth? Where are you working? What are you doing?

Body and Health: How do you feel? What are you doing in your healthy body? Visualize yourself healthy and what you will be doing and feeling. Do not focus on the illness itself. Avoid using words that reference illness.

Relationships and Personal: What is your relationship with your spouse and family like? If you are looking for a relationship, visualize that person's ideal qualities. Who are your friends? What do those friendships feel like? Do you see yourself going back to school, getting training, or growing spiritually? Do you meditate or go on spiritual retreats? Do you want to learn to play an instrument or write a book? What are you doing with your family and friends in the free time you have created for yourself? What hobbies are you pursuing? What kinds of vacations do you take? What do you do for fun?

Once you have your ideal life on the drawing board, take some time to fine tune it. It may take a week or more. Spend a bit of time thinking about it each day. This exercise is not just about what you want to accumulate. It is about how you want to feel. Passion and purpose are a very important part of our ideal lives. Infuse your ideal life with passion and things you love to do. It is worth repeating that accumulating things will not make you happy. Happiness comes from within. The same goes for our health. Our health will not make us happy. We can choose to be happy now. It does not mean we cannot have nice things, and it does not mean we are not working on our health. It is the dichotomy of being able to be happy without them, even though we are working to manifest them.

Activate the Laws of Attraction

Now that you know what your ideal life looks like, it is time to activate the Laws of Attraction by using goal setting and affirmations to bring daily focus to our desires. By setting goals and affirmations, we give ourselves an easy sentence to repeat in order to activate our visions from the Create Your Ideal Life exercise. This daily focus will motivate us to take action.

Turning our visions from the Create Your Ideal Life exercise into goals is the first step in activating the Laws of Attraction. Goals are specific targets you want to reach with a deadline by when you will reach them. When setting goals, it is important to be unattached to the outcome. It is not setting up to allow for failure because we are afraid to fail. It is recognizing that often the universe knows a better way. It is being open to a different path. It is going for the specificity and deadline on the goal but being happy even if it does not happen exactly as our goal is worded. Having this mindset removes the fear of failure. I once had a client set a goal of reaching $500k in sales for the year. This was double her previous year. She made it to $480k. She was upset she did not get there. She got depressed and was mad at herself. She lived in that gap instead of being proud of her achievement. She focused on the missing $20k instead of the extra $230k. Goals help create action steps. Goals help build drive and motivation. Goals should not incapacitate you if you do not reach them. Not reaching a goal in the time set is equally as valuable as reaching it because you have gained more tools in your new achievements to bring you closer to it next time, and you have also learned lessons in why you did not make it.

Personally, I am not a fan of doing a monthly or yearly goal unless the person is totally unattached to outcome. It creates too much stress and becomes a rat race. You get on the hamster wheel of trying to accumulate, nonstop. We are working to heal our bodies, not create more stress. When writing this book, I had a goal to have this book done by the end of the year that I started writing it. This motivated me to write most days. I also was in a state of allowance that it would come to be in its own time. Like all authors, I have a goal for it to be a bestseller. I am also in a state of acceptance if it is not. I learned that writing a book takes a lot of work and money for first time authors. Even if I do not make any profit off it, that is okay. I am writing out of passion and love. I am writing it to be of service. I am writing it to share the tools I have learned that have helped me. If it helps one person, that is enough. It is so important to find joy in the process of achieving our goals, not just be obsessed with the end results.

When I first started writing this book, I was rushing to get it done and would be frustrated if I were interrupted or the words did not come. Frustration, anxiety, or any lower-vibration emotion is a key indicator that you are no longer in touch with source energy. I slowed down and really worked to find the joy in writing, itself. I focused on having gratitude for how when I sit down in a peaceful state, the words just flow out. I just sit down and write, later reading parts and not knowing how I wrote them. If you find yourself anxious, frustrated, or impatient when working on goal setting or any aspect of mindset work, take some time to meditate on the joy and gratitude for the process; work more on letting go of your attachment to the end result.

When I first started in mindset work, my coach had me write a lot of goals. I was very specific and had big goals with short timelines. I made most of them and created some amazing things. It was mind-blowing to see the power of the Laws of Attraction at work. I was very much in stage two consciousness: manifestation. I was also very stressed out working to achieve them. When we went over goals again at *Train the Trainer* with Jack Canfield, I was unable to write a goal. It did not resonate with me. I had just created so much, and I wanted to enjoy it. To just be and allow. To trust the universe. To take what came to me. I still affirmed and visualized, but I trusted it would happen at its own time. That is where I moved for the first time into stage three consciousness: allowance. I have found the ultimate attraction point to be when you are happy where you are, setting goals for the future, in acceptance if they do not happen and in faith that everything works out exactly as it should.

Below are some tools for writing goals. If goal setting does not feel right for you, that is okay, just skip to affirmations and visualizations. If you do not want to set goals, ask yourself if you are happy now. If yes, great. If no, try this process. If you are just avoiding committing because of fear of failure, then you definitely want to work through this process, as we will be tackling that.

There are two types of goals: result goals and process goals. "I want to weigh 140lbs by December 30th" is a result goal. "I will walk one hour every day starting March 30th," is a process goal, as it helps you get to your result goal. Be as specific as possible when writing your goals. Place a deadline on them that will motivate you to take action but not cause intense stress. The difference between a goal and an affirmation is that a goal is a declaration, an objective in the future, an, "I will." An affirmation is present tense, "I am." Affirmations are speaking from the goal being manifested. When setting goals, expect obstacles and fears to appear. Only include things you can control. Do not include other people unless they are working with you in setting and reaching the goal. If you set a goal to be married by a certain time, have a vision of your ideal mate. If you already are engaged and the other person is wanting to get married, by all means include them. If you are not in a relationship, do not include someone who does not want to be married to you into your goal or your vision.

Goal Amounts: Achievable (the smallest you would be happiest with and know you can achieve), Stretch (the next step up that will get you to think outside the box and push you but is not crazy), Leap (you would really have to up level and work hard to reach this). Choose a goal amount in between stretch and leap.

Exercise #18: Set Goals: Write goals for your vision in each area of the previous exercise. Be specific on how much and by when. Include process goals for each result goal in all three categories: Financial and Career, Health and Body, Relationships and Personal.

After creating your goals, the second step in activating the Laws of Attraction is to turn each goal into an affirmation. An affirmation is in the present tense, as if it has already happened. We create the affirmation by using empowering language and gratitude. Our language should be of high vibration and start with the words, "I AM." These powerful words give a command to the subconscious. We use gratitude, as it is one of the most powerful emotions. It puts us in the highest state of vibration. I am so happy and grateful I am [add your goal here in present tense]." Examples:

"I am so proud and grateful I am healthy and full of energy."

"I am so happy and grateful I am detoxifying optimally."

"I am so thankful I easily make $5000 each month."

"I am so grateful I completed my training."

Exercise #19: Create Affirmations: Create affirmations for each of your goals in the three categories. Go over your goals and affirmations once a day to activate the Laws of Attraction.

The third step in activating the Laws of Attraction is to get into action. Just visualizing something is not usually enough to make it happen. I say "usually," as there are some people who are master manifesters, and that is all they need to do. For most of us, goals and affirmations are motivators to take action. Action is telling the universe you trust your vision is coming to you and that you are taking the first step.

Exercise #20: Take Action: Pick three goals that are most important to you, one from each category, and write a list of five action steps you can take to move toward your goals. Make the first action for each goal something you can do in the next day or week. Once you complete those action steps, tackle the remaining goals.

If you find fear of failure is stopping you from acting, remember there is no such thing as failure. There are only lessons. Also, it is okay to lean in and try things. If you are working toward a goal and decide it is not right for you, that is okay, too. That is just new information. Had you not tried, you would not have discovered that you did not like it. Often, we are not allowed to stop something as children. We are labelled as quitters. It is a limiting belief. Trying things and allowing yourself to change your mind is honoring yourself and your connection to source through passion. Make this your new empowering belief.

Another fear that keeps people from acting is fear of criticism and judgment. Both criticism and judgment are just feedback. No matter what you do, you will be judged. You could be the most beautiful, perfect person in the world, and someone would find a fault. There is a saying, "If you are afraid of judgment, do not be seen, just stay home." The truth is you would get judged for that, too.

Feedback is critical to tell us if we are on or off track toward our goals. Look at it as a tool for growth. Once you begin to act, you will start getting feedback about whether you are doing it right. You will get data, advice, help, suggestions, direction, and criticism that will help you move forward toward your goal. All feedback gives you new knowledge and tools, if you can learn to not take it as a personal attack. How you respond to feedback can make all the difference in how successful you are at achieving your goals. All actions do not work. It is important to get feedback as to why. Most people get defensive, ignore feedback, get angry, cry, get depressed, break down, or give up when they get feedback. The smart way to respond is to stop and listen to the feedback, adjust what you are doing if it makes sense, then try again.

Another fear that prevents action is the fear of rejection. When we start to take action, we often have to ask for help. One of the hardest words we hear is "no." It can trigger a lot of emotions. *Go for No* by Andrea Waltz and Richard Fenton was a life-changing book for me. It helped me create my business. Do not count your "yesses" and stop when you reach your goal. Start counting your "nos," Expect them, seek them out, and get really comfortable with them. Every time you hear the word "no," ask for feedback as to why not. If you get rejected, keep trying. When you do not take the rejection personally, you will be able to ask freely. If emotions do come up, it is a gift. It means you have some inner work to do. Ask yourself, "If I had the confidence and did not care what people thought of me, what would I do?" Those are your first steps. That is where growth lies. That is what you need to do.

Using these tools will help you achieve your goals by activating the Laws of Attraction and by lighting a fire under you to get motivated into action. First, get clear about what you desire, then use goal setting and affirmations to create your inspiration to act. Then, start getting into action every day to move toward your goal.

Empathy

Empathy is a skill. Most people are not born with it. Many people will say they are empaths, but what they call empathy is not true empathy, and it certainly is not healthy. I remember on Facebook, there was a video going around about empaths. The little stick person empath was going about their day, and every person they would meet would hug them or tell them about their problems, and this would drain the empath's energy. The other person would go away feeling better while leaving the empath progressively depleted. This is not empathy.

Empathy is not taking and holding onto someone's pain while giving them your energy. Empathy is imagining what other people are thinking and experiencing, so you can understand them, and they can feel felt. You are providing a space for them to express their emotions. Empathy is validating their feelings and their experience while suspending your own thoughts and feelings. Before being able to show empathy, you want to get in touch with your own emotions. If you are numb or repressing emotions because you have been told to suck it up as a child, you will want to address this first. Showing vulnerability is also a skill. If you are easily triggered by other people's emotions, it is important to work on those triggers first. It will be impossible to show empathy if you are unable to stay in the present moment.

Let us look at what empathy is not. Empathy is not sympathizing, saying, "I am so sorry for you. That is so sad." Empathy is not one-upping or comparing: "Last week this happened to me," or, "These people have it much worse," or, "You should be thankful for this." There is a time and place to use tools like gratitude and looking at the grand scheme of things, but it is not the place in acute trauma. If someone is asking for help when they are stuck, that is the time to offer solutions and tools.

Empathy is not taking on the other person's problems, staying in their shoes past the time of connection, taking on their energy, or bearing their trauma. There needs to be a barrier on energy. Empathy is best given when the empath is in a high-vibrational state and has good skills in protecting their energy. Review the "Protect Your Energy" section for more tools on this. It is very important to develop skills in protecting your energy if you are put into situations where you are required to show empathy on a regular basis. No amount of you feeling sadness, anger, or other emotions will make the other person's suffering or problems better. When you become a beacon of light, your higher energy will help them feel better without draining you. It is all about giving from abundance. If you are not at this level yet, it is best to limit the time spent around people in lower-vibration states so that it does not have a detrimental effect on your health and wellbeing.

Now we will look at what empathy is. Empathy is learning to listen and to send the ego to the backseat while listening. Empathy is connection without judgment or offering solutions. Empathy is joining and feeling another's emotions, while remaining separate.

Empathy is easier to provide to our children once we are able to remove ourselves from our past triggers, as children usually move quickly from one emotion to the next. You are also less likely to experience energy draining from their intense emotion over dropping their ice cream cone. For adults, our kids' problems are not as emotionally draining as the problems of other adults.

Having a safe place to express emotions is a basic need for everyone. This is critical for childhood development. When kids experience something like getting injured, bullying, jealousy, etc., parents will more often undermine what they are going through and tell them, "It is alright, you are fine," or, "Suck it up, that is part of life," or, "No one likes a cry baby," or, "It is not a big deal," etc. Their emotions are dismissed. Parents are too often focused on a behavior and teaching lessons and skills. As parents, we want to allow our kids to have their emotions. We want to allow them to move through their emotions and validate them. Connect, show empathy, and allow your child to feel their emotions.

If you never received empathy from your parents, when you meet someone who allows you to express yourself without judgment, it brings connection, warmth, comfort, and peace. It helps you feel whole and complete. Providing empathy in your relationships will help bring them to a new level. Empathy is listening to understand. Empathy is not listening to respond or fix.

This is something that I work on. As a coach, people hire me to help them find solutions. I have learned that friends and family do not necessarily want you to offer them advice. They just want to have someone listen. When I first learned about taking responsibility for my life, this was also tough for me. Seeing someone complaining and attracting more of the same would shift me into fix mode. It is something I work on, to just allow the people in my life to be who they are and accept it is their responsibility to want to change. Until they want to change on their own, they will not hear any message. It is possible to plant a seed, but it is up to them as adults to take the responsibility for themselves. Empathy is best for acute trauma. When someone is constantly complaining or stuck in a trauma about the same issue for weeks, months, or even years, empathy is not the best choice. Changing the subject and shifting focus is much better so that it shifts their attraction point. Sometimes I will ask, "Do you want me to just listen, or would you like some coaching on the issue, as you seem to be stuck?" This can help shed some awareness on how they are stuck and may need help. It is up to them when they are ready to work on it.

When empathizing, we want to focus on our body language, not our words. The right brain connects with touch and emotion. The left, logical brain connects with words. If you are close to the person, holding them, hugging them, or placing a hand on them are all great options. If you are not close to the person, just sit with them. Use compassionate facial expressions and connect at their level. When a person has calmed, you can offer comforting phrases like, "That must really be hard," "I am here for you," and, "It's okay to feel that way."

Saying, "I understand," is not always best as they may feel you do not really understand because you have not felt something similar. We do not want to shift focus from them onto you. It is okay to say nothing at all. Just be there and listen actively. Put your phone down. Stay focused and listen intently, without judgment or comparison. Remember that feelings come and go. Feelings do not define a person. Be open minded and in a state of allowance. Let go of how you think the situation should be.

Conscious Parenting

Even if you are not a parent or do not plan on becoming one, this is still a very important section for a few reasons. Most of our limiting beliefs come from our childhood, and most of those come from our very own parents. Looking at the science behind developmental parenting and understanding the brain as it grows will allow you to repair your past trauma and help you identify your limiting beliefs so you can create empowering ones. The more you discover about parenting, the more you discover and understand about yourself and why you are who you are.

The second reason why this section is important for everyone is that of all the books I have read and the courses I have taken, the ones on conscious parenting have been the most helpful to develop my communication skills. Honestly, the time I have spent on this subject has done more for my relationships with my husband and family than anything else I have done. If our goal is peace and joy, this is a very important skill to develop.

The third reason this is a must-read section is that it will help you relate to and feel compassion for the young children that come into your life. It also helps bring compassion to your own parents and other people in your life when you recognize how their pasts have shaped who they are today.

If you are a parent, learning about conscious parenting will allow you to prevent a lot of the trauma and limiting beliefs you have from developing in your child or children. Sadly, many people do not ever come to the conscious awareness to do this mindset training and are left suffering their entire lives. This is why conscious parenting is so important. Conscious parenting helps raise conscious children, who are resilient and can adapt to stress. These children can communicate and express their emotions in healthy ways. They follow their passion and purpose and are filled with empowering beliefs. The most important part of all is that conscious parenting will help you develop a strong relationship with your child. Becoming a conscious parent will really help bring peace into your household. Peace is needed to heal.

If you are thinking of becoming a parent in the future, putting this knowledge in place ahead of time will make your journey as a parent much easier right off the bat. Though this is a big section, it is just an introduction to conscious parenting. I would recommend diving deep into this subject if you currently have children or are thinking of having children. There are many great books and courses out there. Some of my favorite authors are Dan Siegel, Deborah MacNamara, Shefali Tsabary, Susan Stiffelman, Lawrence J Cohen, and Janet Lansbury. I highly recommend investing in Dr. Gordon Neufeld's online courses.

For most of history, parenting has been based on dominance. Parents are the boss, and kids need to behave a certain way. Control is the key in dominant parenting, "Do what I say because I say so," or, "Do what I say because society says that it is best." Kids are only loved if they are good, or at least that is how they see it. There is a false sense of respect based on fear. The child's feelings do not matter, and children are seen as manipulative to get attention. Children are expected to behave even if the parent is not modeling those same skills that they want in their children.

Kids growing up with this type of parenting do not have the ability or opportunity to express their emotions. They do not have the ability to defend their emotional rights. Kids go into survival mode, and emotional trauma will live in their subconscious and affect their ability to thrive. Reward-based and consequence-based parenting are also about controlling behavior. It just uses a nicer label. As kids get older, it gets increasingly more difficult to find consequences and rewards. Once the power is gone, you have nothing left. You never learn to influence them. Kids will focus on how mean you are instead of on a lesson when you use consequences or punishments to try to change their behavior. This damages your relationship with them.

Conscious parenting is about taking everything you have learned on mindfulness and putting it to action in parenting. Conscious parenting is not permissive parenting. There are still boundaries and limits. Conscious parenting is about valuing our relationships with our children above all else. It is about treating them as equals and teaching them their voices matter. They deserve to be heard. Conscious parenting is about letting go of our expectations of how our children should be and shifting focus from behavior to connection and emotion.

Conscious parenting is deciding what skills you want your child to have and then modeling them, yourself. Children are great spiritual teachers and show us where we need to do more work. Conscious parenting is about teaching children skills they will need to thrive as they become developmentally capable of learning them. It is done with patience, empathy, and flexibility. Conscious parenting is about teaching emotional intelligence and empowerment. Coercion, shame, time-outs, manipulation, bribes, and threats are all wounding to our children and are not needed.

Parents frequently end up trying to live vicariously through their kids, seeing their children's successes as their own, instead of allowing their children to find their own success based on their inner passions, joy, and fulfillment. In conscious parenting, we let go of expectations on our children and recognize where our egos are looking for approval from others based on how our children behave. Relationship trumps behavior in conscious parenting. Whenever you see a behavior from your child that you do not like, it means your child has a need that is not being met or has a skill that still needs to be learned. Focus on your child's needs. More often than not, a child's brain is not developed enough to perform the skill you want them to know. No amount of punishments, consequences, or time-outs will make your child's brain mature faster. All it will do is damage your relationship and put a stop to brain growth. Our children's brains cannot develop when they are being wounded. A healthy relationship with you where they are free to feel and express emotions is what is needed for your child's brain to grow.

In dominant parenting, children learn to please others but not themselves. When they grow up, they do the same. They become people-pleasers, put themselves last, and are often depressed. Dominant parenting creates limiting beliefs of not being enough, not being good, not being seen, and not feeling important. This happens often when children are pushed by parents to be the best in school and go to college for something that will bring prestige and money instead of joy and purpose. Do not impose an academic career on your child that he or she is not passionate about. Develop a wide array of interests and pursuits. Make time for unstructured play and just being together without an agenda.

During Kaiden's first summer knowing how to walk, I wanted to go on adventures because I love to play and have fun. I had an expectation that Kaiden should love the same. We would go adventuring together. I bought him things that I thought would be fun, like swings, wagons, and things to ride on. Kaiden had other ideas. He was more reserved and needed time to build confidence. I had a moment of frustration when he did not want to go in the swing. Luckily, I recognized my ego wanting to live through him and what I thought was right. That left us both unhappy. I shifted back to allowing him to gain confidence. Now he is bold and brave because I gave him the time to develop at his own pace. This is something tiny, but it happens all the time in various degrees. As parents, we push our kids into sports, academics, and even college courses based on what we think is best for them. They are born with an "emotional guidance system," as Abraham Hicks calls it in the *Teachings of Abraham*. Allow them to get in touch with and follow it. When they are in touch with their emotional guidance system, they are following their passions and purposes.

When we use praise to manipulate behavior, we are saying, "I love you when you do good things." It is great to praise your child, as long as you are also showing equal love and approval for them as they are, even when they do things you do not like. Conscious parenting says, "I am here to love and support you no matter what." Whining, tantrums, meltdowns, and strong emotions are not bad and do not need to be turned off or avoided. They are all a healthy part of learning to express emotions. I like to affirm to myself, "Express your feelings, my child. I will model calmness, adaptation, patience, compassion, and resilience. As you grow, I will help you learn these skills, knowing it will take time and patience while your brain develops. For now, I will be the space for you to express your emotions."

Exercise #21: Your Childhood Needs: Think back to when you were a child. What was it that you truly wanted from your parents? Take a few minutes to write down what your needs were. How were they met, and how were they not met?

For most, what we wanted was a safe place. A place with boundaries and structure. A place where we had unconditional love, approval, and acceptance. Conscious parenting is based on creating secure attachment. This is where a child has at least one caregiver meeting their attachment needs. Yes, attachment is a need. Attachment equals survival. If a baby mammal did not attach to a caregiver, it would not survive. Secure attachment leads to being taken care of. When we see attachment as the most important need and that it is hardwired into our brains for survival, it changes how we look at our children and their behavior.

Many people think attachment is just baby bonding. It may start out as that, but as children grow, their attachment deepens as their brain develops. Children need to be near you and also need to feel that they are loved unconditionally, that you know them, that they can trust you, and that they belong. Kids need to feel accepted for who they are, not what they do. They need to feel you have their backs and will not shame them. They need to feel special and important. They need to be seen and heard. "I see you. I am here no matter what. I will take care of you. You are safe. You are loved. I will meet your needs." All of these are what create secure attachment.

We want to go over and above, filling our children's attachment cups until they are overflowing. If you were provided with every meal, you may not feel hungry, but if you were worried the next meal might not come, you would always be focusing on food. Give your children a feast of attachment so they know they will never go hungry. This way, they can put their energy into growth instead of looking for more attachment. In the "Protect Your Energy" section, you learned to create an energetic barrier around yourself. Children are not capable of doing this for themselves. Secure attachment provides this shield for them, and it helps keep them safe from emotional wounding.

Even if you have not been using this approach with your child, it is never too late to start. Attachment can be built at any age. Adults who did not receive secure attachment as children and are feeling the wounding of their childhood can use the "Healing the Past Meditation" in "Part Three: Spirit" to help heal those wounds. As adults, cultivating attachment with our children, spouses, friends, and family will meet those needs now.

When children are securely attached, childhood is a fun time of learning and exploration. It is about discovering oneself. Children are not meant to look for love. If a child does not receive secure attachment, they will start to seek it out from other people. They may try to find it in a loving stranger who they feel is meeting their needs, or they may look for it in their peers. When their attachment needs are ignored, they will look for them to be filled elsewhere.

I highly recommend reading *Hold onto Your Kids* by Dr. Gordon Neufeld, as it demonstrates how most children in today's world have become peer-attached due to lack of attachment with parents and caregivers. It goes in depth into the issues this is creating for our children. If you have a child you believe is peer-attached or is displaying behaviors like aggression, anxiety, depression, social media addiction, or gaming addiction, Dr. Neufeld's courses dive deep into how to reconnect with your child and heal. They are a great place to start, as is seeing a practitioner who specializes in his developmental approach. When looking for a practitioner or therapist, make sure they are true developmentalists. Many may be labelled as developmental but have a background in the learning theory, which is all about controlling behavior versus getting to the root cause.

Sadly, childhood has become a time of high anxiety as kids try to meet expectations set on them by parents and society. Instead, childhood should be a time of free development and exploration. Kids feel oppressed and overwhelmed. We become more invested in doing instead of being. School, lessons, sports, homework: every ounce of space is booked. Get in the moment and see what your child needs. Ask, "Is this for me or for my child?" You can have money, prestige, and a career but remain lost on who you are and what brings you joy.

How your parents parented you will affect how you are parenting your child. The times you did not get the secure attachment you needed have created trauma and limiting beliefs about who you are. Those traumas can cause you to be triggered by your child's behaviors, and in turn, you will react with very strong emotions. It is important to go over your past and create an integrated life story. Life stories that have not been made sense of can limit us as parents and in our lives in general, and they can cause us to pass down the same painful trauma that was passed down to us. Doing just the opposite of your parents will not fix the problem, either. Kids live through whatever we are experiencing. Uncovering the cause of triggers and making sense of them is the way to end the cycle.

Exercise #22: Your Parenting Past: Reflect and integrate your memories into your sense of self. Create a story of your childhood. Go over any painful or traumatic events that are readily available for you to access in your memory and look for lessons and how they helped you grow spiritually. If this brings up too much emotion, it is best to work with a coach or therapist who can help you process these issues.

Besides the exercise above, another way to discover past trauma is to look at where you are triggered with your children or even with other adults. We have talked about how we have implicit memories that are not integrated in the brain; these can be triggered and cause us to react in extreme ways to normal situations. Often, they are buried deep in our subconscious mind. If your child does something, and you react with big emotions, the odds are you have been triggered by a past trauma. For example, if your child does not listen, you may get very angry because you did not feel you had a voice as a child. This can cause you to react harshly. You may react exactly as your parent did, or you may get upset with your child because they are showing more courage than you did by standing up for themselves. All these emotions surface from your past and are then directed at your child. Another example is when your child cries. It brings up sadness from when you were neglected as a child. You may then get incredibly stressed every time your child cries and need to rush in immediately to comfort your younger self, which you are projecting onto your child.

Having extreme emotion after a small event, being out of control, or patterns of reactions are good indications you have been triggered. Recognize it is not about your kids. It is about the healing you need to do. Be the author of your life. Go over your life story and make sense of it and how it makes you who you are. Be aware of how your limiting beliefs developed and transform them into empowering ones. Go through traumas and integrate them in a healthy way.

Exercise #23: Recognizing and Working Through Triggers: Name a reaction you do not like that you have toward your kids. What characteristic or trait in your child do you have trouble dealing with? Do you do something similar, or are you the opposite? Did your parents do something similar or opposite? How did that make you feel? How did you cope with it? What did you think about yourself? What limiting belief did you create? How has this affected you? How could you turn this thought around? What would your higher self say to this belief or thought? Go back in time to when this happened. What would you have said to your parent(s) about what you needed? What do you think your parent needed at the time? What would your parent's soul say to your younger self? How will you create better communication with your own child based on what your younger self needed? What does your child need? What skills do they need to work on? What can you learn from your child's behavior?

When looking at your past parenting and transitioning to conscious parenting, let go of guilt about how you used to parent. You were doing the best you could with the tools you had at the time. Be proud and kind to yourself. It is not parenting for perfection. It is a learning process, and you are here now trying to make changes.

A big part of conscious parenting is setting up boundaries and values. Boundaries and family values should be set up with parents and children together, if children are old enough to share ideas. Values will be individual to each family. Get together as a family and write them down. Put them where everyone can see them.

Examples of values are: We treat everyone kindly. We are open to new ideas. We listen when someone is speaking. We apologize and make things better. We keep our house clean. We love each other unconditionally. We have fun every day. We respect each other's personal space.

Boundaries and limits are put into place to keep children safe and teach skills. They need to be developmentally suited to each child. They are meant to satisfy basic human needs. They do prevent misbehavior because we teach them to do the right thing. Remember, if a child is not developmentally capable of a behavior, lose the expectation that it is going to happen. It takes a long time for their frontal lobe to develop. A child who has been through a lot of wounding will take even longer. If a child is not capable of a behavior, it is the adult's responsibility to change their environment or situation to make it safe for them. If an eight-year-old is hitting at recess, it is not their behavior that needs to change. The adults in his life need to realize he is unable to handle recess at this time. The adults need to see the lack of maturity and change his situation without shaming him. Perhaps have him help out in another class at recess. In order for the brain to grow, a child needs attachment. An eight-year-old hitting indicates his parents need to work on reconnecting with their child and healing the wounds he has been experiencing. They need to reduce peer interaction and reduce the separation between them and their child.

Rules are inflexible and implement fear, punishment, and control. Rules leave no space for empathy and connection. Boundaries leave room for compromise and flexibility. Boundaries provide structure. Boundaries include: holding hands when crossing the street, bedtime, dinner time, curfews, menus, etc. When a boundary needs to be upheld, and the child is pushing against it, first connect and show empathy. Listen to their feelings. Once calm, explain why it is there. Offer choices, if possible. Sometimes, a boundary just has to stick. Enforce it and allow them to express their feelings of anger and sadness. Show empathy and stick to what needs to be done. For example, if you have a designated time for technology, and when it is time to put it away, they argue. You can respond by removing the technology, listening to their frustration, and showing you understand how they feel. Explain why you have the boundary and stick to it. Allow them to be upset and feel their feelings. The only way they can work through an emotion is to feel and express it. If your child is full of frustration and is acting with aggression, recognize that it needs to come out. Help them find a safe way to express their frustration instead of trying to stop it. Trying to stop a behavior is like trying to plug a volcano. It will erupt. Say to your child, "I see you are frustrated. Let me help you express that in a safe way."

In one of my favorite books, *Parenting Without Power Struggles*, Susan Stiffelman uses the best analogy I have ever read to explain how a parent can get a child to follow them without needing punishment or fear. She explains that a parent wants to be the captain of their ship. If you were on a cruise ship, you would want a strong, calm, confident captain, one who does not lose themselves when a stressful situation happens. If you were on a ship and your captain had an adult meltdown over a storm, you would quickly lose confidence in your captain's abilities to be in command. You want a captain who can weather the storms calmly. To be the captain of your ship, you will have to do the same. Calmly and confidently weather your child's emotions and the events that come to you in life. Take charge, set boundaries and limits, and maintain them when necessary. Be flexible and listen. Be resilient and adapt. More often than not, parents get into a power struggle with their kids and argue about limits and boundaries. Doing this causes you to lose your captaincy and end up on equal grounds. When you completely lose your cool because of your child's behavior, your child is now the captain of your ship. You are showing them that their behavior has power over you. See your child's behavior as a challenge to stay peaceful instead of something that is stressful.

Emotional maturity is not something you can force on a child. Even if you explain something to your child and feel they understood, that does not mean they will be able to access that in the moment. Behavioral parenting has led parents to believe they can force maturity on a child through rewards and punishment. This is not true. The child is not mature when this technique is used; they are only holding back their feelings. This is why communication skills are not common in adults. At different ages of development, children become able to process their emotions. They require a guide to properly teach them. A two-year-old is not capable of reasoning and reflecting on emotions due to their brain development. They cannot even name their emotions at age two. As children grow, they develop emotional abilities with the help of an adult to manage them. The first step in development is to express their emotions. Joy, anger, jealousy, sadness, etc., all need to be felt and expressed. Young kids tend to do this in a very big fashion through screams of joy to tantrums of frustration. These are all normal development. Do not squash their expression of joy or frustration. Our adult brains find this expression uncomfortable, mostly because we were likely punished for our expressions as children. Allowing kids to feel and express their emotions is the first step in processing them and integrating events into a healthy life story. As they get older, children begin to be able to name emotions with assistance from their caregivers. As they develop more, they are able to think about and reflect on their emotions.

If a child is only able to express their emotions but is unable to name them, we need to give them a safe place to do this without being triggered, ourselves. Toddlers have big emotions they cannot control. As adults, all we can do is connect, show empathy, and allow their upset to turn from frustration to sadness and then acceptance. To them, what they are feeling is very important, and they can only think about one thing at a time. We do not want to distract or redirect them too much, otherwise they will not be able to feel their feelings and express them. If you always try to stop them from expressing their emotions, they also will not learn the process of moving from anger to sadness to acceptance. Dr. Neufeld calls this "The Wall of Futility." When a child realizes they are not going to get their way, they can move to sadness and grieve for the loss. After that, they can move to acceptance. This process is called adaptation, and it is a key part of brain development that leads to resilience as adults. If children are not able to move through frustration to sadness, then adaptation will not develop; as an adult, the person will not be able to handle stress and loss. When adults are able to stay calm in a tantrum or meltdown, children can move through it, and their brains can grow.

When I first learned about this, I realized whenever Kaiden was getting upset, we tended to redirect him to something else. When we would hold our boundary of no, he would get angry, and we would respond by moving him or showing him something else to do. While it is okay to redirect sometimes, we do want our children to experience not getting their way. Eric and I were uncomfortable with full-blown tantrums and still wanted to prevent the behavior. This led to Kaiden progressively getting angrier. Eventually, redirecting stopped working. He also had not experienced moving from anger to sadness very often, so he ended up getting stuck in anger for a long time. He started to hit and bite because he had so much built-up frustration. When I understood this, I realized I had to work on my discomfort around his tantrums and allow him to move through his emotions. The next time we went for a walk in minus fifteen degrees Celsius provided the opportunity. He did not want to wear his mittens and kept taking them off. I upheld the boundary, and each time he took them off, I put them back on. He went into full tantrum, complete with kicking, screaming, and pinching. It would have been so easy to bring him back to the van and go home. We did this for twenty minutes before he hit "The Wall of Futility," and his anger turned to sadness. He cried for five minutes. I stayed calm the entire time, not trying to end the tantrum, just allowing it, and holding my boundary. I kept myself safe by preventing his hits and kicks with my hands. When he moved to sadness, I comforted him in a warm embrace. Then he was fine and ready to play. Each tantrum after that lasted less and less time. When I see he is starting to get frustrated a lot, I know he needs to find his tears. Since we started to hold boundaries and allow his feelings, his hitting and biting have stopped. Now, when something does not go his way, he gets a bit upset, finds his tears, and looks for us to give him a big hug. Then he moves on. How many people do you know who cannot let go of anger and resentment? A big contributor to this was not having the space as a child to move through these stages without judgment or punishment.

The key for the adult is to recognize any thoughts they have around a tantrum. They may feel that a tantrum makes them a bad parent, or a tantrum is bad. Recognize any anger brewing. Take deep breaths, remind yourself that it is natural and healthy, and show empathy for your child's emotions. One thing that worked well for Kaiden when he was hitting was, "It looks like you are really mad, and your hands want to hit; you can hit this pillow." Getting the frustration out is needed. Stopping the hitting will just lead to displacement onto a sibling, animal, or themselves. Allow them to hit in a safe way. In time, as their brain develops, it will stop. They will learn to use words when you narrate their feelings. Just acknowledging and showing empathy can often stop the tantrum. Check your stories about hitting and biting. Check how you are projecting into the future your ten-year-old still biting or your teen hitting. Stay present and realize, at this time, it is normal development. Allow their expression of emotions to occur safely, and model calmness.

As toddlers gain more language, adults can begin to name what their toddlers are feeling. As they get older, they will learn to use words to express what they are feeling instead of outbursts of anger. Yelling and hitting will turn into, "I am so mad!" Children go through a shift around age five to seven, where their frontal lobe undergoes huge development and is capable of integrative functioning. For some kids, it does not happen until seven to nine years old. This switch is also not guaranteed to happen at all. If a child experiences too much trauma, brain development can stop. Many adults do not have well developed integration because of this. During this shift, children start to be able to feel more than one emotion at once. Before this, the limbic system in their brain, responsible for emotions, could only send one emotion into their prefrontal cortex at a time. Let that sink in for a moment. Before this shift, your child is not capable of feeling two emotions at a time. When this shift occurs, they will begin to be able to mix emotions together. To feel angry at you and feel their love for you at the same time will give them the ability to not hit. Strong emotions are hard to mix and will take longer. In time, children begin to be able to reason, reflect on what they are feeling, and express their emotions in a safe way through words. This all takes place with an adult modeling the behavior for them and guiding them through their experiences. Think of times in your life as an adult when you have been upset and had outbursts of yelling or crying. It is a good indication that you need some work on these skills, too. The same will happen with your children. Even when you feel they have learned the skill, suddenly, they are having a meltdown. This is all normal. You still have adult meltdowns. You may feel you have more to melt down about, but to a child, what they feel is very important. Remember those times you lose control so you can show empathy.

Children who were not allowed to express their emotions as children and were punished for doing so, often grow into adults who hold in their emotions because they fear conflict. The opposite of expression is depression, and not being able to safely communicate how you feel will lead to many relationship issues. Learning to allow yourself to feel your emotions, reflect, and properly express what is bothering you will bring a new level of peace and joy to your life. Mindset training is not just about turning around thoughts. It is learning to express how you feel in a safe way.

122

Kids being defiant and saying "no" is needed for them to develop their sense of self. Frustration and defiance are big milestones in brain development. This happens significantly in the so called "terrible twos." Securely attached children will begin to say "no" to everything that is not their idea and want to do everything themselves. When you see their behavior as healthy maturation, it becomes amusing. Now that I understand healthy development, it brings me laughter instead of frustration when I ask Kaiden if he wants to go downstairs and he says, "No," then a moment later heads downstairs. Using discipline to try to stop this maturation only leads to more frustration which only leads to more meltdowns. Separation-based discipline like time-outs, taking away something they love, or emotional withdrawal says, "You only love me when I behave a certain way." It is easy to see why people grow up putting their needs last and trying to please others. Separation-based discipline hurts attachment and is very wounding. Teach your children that they are loved with all emotions. Every emotion is welcome. You can take care of them all. Quality of attachment with caregivers develops kids' emotional skills. Without connection, the brain shuts down to protect itself and maturation halts.

Very young children live moment to moment. They experience, then let things go. The harder part is for adults to do the same. Do not hold resentment for children's past behavior, and do not label them. For older children, once they are calm, you can have them reflect on what they felt, name how they felt, and go over other ways they can express their emotions. Do not expect them to develop the tools right away. Allow them to make suggestions, instead of just lecturing on what you want to see. Often, lessons may not happen until a later time in the day or not at all if their brain is not developed enough to do so. That is okay, too. Ask your child to tell a story through play (drawing, toys, or stories) to help integrate it into their brain in a healthy way. Always remember your relationship trumps behavior and lessons. Learning comes through brain development.

Allowing kids to express their emotions can be messy. Society does not like it, and you will get all sorts of advice. When Kaiden used to bite me when people were around, I would often hear, "I would not let him do that. He needs to be punished. Bite him back." When he bites or pinches, it sometimes can put me into reaction mode, but it is my job to model to him that we do not meet violence with violence. It is my job to model calmness. He has since stopped biting. The biting phase did not last long because I did not react to it. Developmental neuroscience shows us that children being allowed to express and work through their emotions is what is needed to create an emotionally stable individual. Emotional tension will not release until it is expressed. If you stop it, it will come up elsewhere and often more intensely.

If your child can instantly stop a tantrum, the child is using their upper brain. In this situation, calmly give realistic, firm boundaries and implement them. A lower brain tantrum is a loss of control and requires comfort. This is almost always the case with younger children. If the child is truly out of control in a tantrum and may be violent, hold them close and remove them from the scene. Let go of pressure and judgment from others and protect your child's dignity. Our brains perceive pain as a threat, so when they are hitting or biting you, you immediately activate the stress response and fight or flight. Staying calm takes practice. Spanking, yelling, or time alone shifts focus away from their behavior and onto yours; how mean, unfair, and uncaring you are. All of these punishments hurt attachment and wound the child. It creates a cortisol response, which prevents learning and brain growth. All of these punishments activate the lower brain and cause it to be more dominant. Instead, use a time-in. Withdraw together to a safe place and move through the emotions.

Sometimes as parents, we lose control and make mistakes. These are also times for growth and opportunities to learn. Learn to recognize when you are losing control. Close your mouth and remove yourself. Collect yourself. Protect your child. Get control and model self-regulation. Then, repair whatever harm has been done. Apologize, accept responsibility, retell the story, and listen to their feelings. Have an empowered conversation. Start with your intention, take responsibility for your part, then state your feelings and needs in "I" statements. Do not mirror what they say, as that is frustrating. Try to connect with them. Do not try to fix everything. Conflict is an opportunity for growth, skill building, learning, and brain development, especially for us. It's okay to miss teachable moments, and it is okay that we still make mistakes in parenting. The goal is to have the intention to be conscious.

Kids may need to talk to someone else after a conflict. Do not embarrass kids in front of people. It takes focus from the lesson you want to teach and again, just makes you seem mean. Shaming hurts attachment and is severely wounding. For parenting mistakes, only listen to your inner critic long enough to gain insight and awareness. Be gentle with yourself. Calmness and connection need to follow conflict.

There is a misconception that attention and connection is spoiling. Love, connection, attention, and time are all needs. You cannot spoil a child by loving them too much or giving them too much of yourself. You cannot spoil a baby by holding it too much or responding to its needs. Spoiling happens when giving a child a sense of entitlement to everything they want and getting it right away, as well as doing everything for them. It also includes sheltering or overprotecting. Never saying "no" and never upholding boundaries prevents a child from learning adaptation skills and is a form of spoiling.

Tips and Exercises for Conscious Parenting

Often, when our children say mean or disrespectful things, our egos get triggered. We think, and sometimes say, "How dare you speak to me like that. You need to show respect." Learn to recognize your ego. Instead of getting upset with undesirable language and saying things that can be harmful, ask your child to try again. Say, "I understand you are upset. Can you ask me again using respectful language?"

When kids do something wrong, healthy reflection comes from getting them to think about how other people feel, not from punishment or shaming. After a conflict, connect with your child. Even if they have done something to hurt someone, they are hurt, also. Connect with them until they calm down. Ask them what happened. Ask them why they behaved the way they did. Listen without judgment. Ask them how they think the other person felt and ask them how they can make it right. Respect them enough to listen to them, and value their contribution to problem-solving. This process only works for children who have made the five to seven shift mentioned earlier. Remember, just because they have reached the age does not mean the development has happened.

The desire to share is not a skill that can be forced. It comes from brain development and does not start to happen until age five. Young children cannot understand that a toy will come back. They are only able to feel one emotion at a time, and all they feel is loss. Forcing a child to share tells them that their needs do not matter. They end up feeling deprived and in need. This does not bring feelings of being generous. It does the opposite. It also creates resentment toward the adult and other child, and it leads to limiting beliefs of not being valuable. It also leads to them becoming people-pleasing adults who always put their own needs last. Recognize your own feelings of being judged by other adults when your child does not share. If another child wants your child's toy, explain to your child that the other child wants to play with the toy when your child is finished. Drop the pressure to share. Empathize with the other child who wants the toy. Acknowledge their frustration and remind them they can play with it when your child is done. This teaches delayed gratification and builds adaptation skills. Waiting is hard. It is also a needed skill. You can redirect the other child with other toys. When your child is done, give it to the other child. It is common that your child may then want it back. Be firm that they were done and can have it back when the other child is finished. As children get older, you can have both of them state how they feel and try to help them problem-solve, if possible. It is still important to respect the choice of the child who had the toy first. Redirect the other child. Later, have some conversations about sharing and empathy with the child who does not want to share. Do this without shaming the child for not sharing. Allow a child to have toys that are theirs only. A toy may not seem valuable to you, but it is to your child. It is like when someone buys a new car. They may not want to let anyone else drive it for a long time. They want to protect it. We allow adults this boundary on their possessions, yet we do not give children the same respect.

Proactive parenting is the best. Try to read cues and prevent behavior before it happens. When you see a behavior that is going to cause problems, try to describe what you see instead of preaching what you want. "I see toys left out; we really value a clean house as a family. Can you put those away?" versus, "Why did you leave your toys out again? I have to remind you over and over. You are such a slob." Another example is, "Your sister looks sad. What do you think is bothering her? How could you help cheer her up?" versus, "Go play with your sister," or, "You need to go and cheer her up." Let children choose. Call attention to behavior and give them the option to help. If you know your child cannot handle a situation, it is best to not put them into it.

Children thrive on routines and structure, especially young children. When a routine is established, if you are getting resistance in ending a task, shifting focus to the next part of the routine will often dissipate the frustration. Ending something fun is a big frustration for children. Kids younger than five to seven are able to hold only one emotion at a time, so we can use this to quell a tantrum before it starts by moving focus to excitement for the next task. When Kaiden does not want to get out of the bath, I shift focus to flushing the toilet. He loves to flush the toilet, and it is the next step after he gets out of the tub.

Share your emotions. This models insight and communication skills. If you say you are happy, and your body language says you are sad, children will be confused by your messages and model what you do. Emotions are good; feel them. Do not share your emotions about your child with your child. Not only is that wounding to the child, but it causes you to lose your captaincy. Your child needs to feel that you can handle anything they throw at you.

Teach self-care and self-compassion. Self-care is essential when raising children. When we are angry, sad, depressed, or resentful, it means our needs are not being met. We need exercise, self-care, time alone, appreciation, help, and empathy just like our children do. Practice self-compassion by being kind to yourself. Allow low-vibration feelings without spiraling out of control. Recognize and teach that failures do not exist; there are only learning experiences. Model this with your actions. Create a shame-free zone in your house so children can try things without fear. Do things you love to do. Make time for your passions. Redefine success to mean focusing on your internal compass, not on other people's expectations. Realize that we as parents are always changing and learning.

Engage their higher brain. Teach your children how their brains work. Ask them what part of the brain they are using. Try to tap into the higher brain during a challenging issue. "You look like you feel angry," brings awareness to feelings. Ask them to negotiate and find other solutions. Avoid always solving problems for them. Resist rescuing if you know they can handle it. Talk about what is right and wrong, instead of preaching. Offer hypothetical situations and ask them how they would act. This helps shape how they make decisions. Model honesty, generosity, kindness, and respect.

Teach skills to keep calm. Teach meditation and breathing techniques from a young age. Teach them how to refocus on gratitude. An easy meditation for kids is to have them lie down and focus on each object in the room. Bring awareness to how they are able to shift their focus. Have them close their eyes. Ask them what they hear. Have them then focus on their breathing. Say you will be quiet while they focus on their breath. Tell them when their mind wanders to move back to focusing on their breath. You can also teach them how to visualize calm, happy places. Bring a period of stillness into each day.

Teach children how to integrate memories through storytelling. Have children tell you stories about their day, stressful events, or emotional traumas. If they are unable to do this, help by telling them stories. Using play, drawing, and acting can all be helpful. Play a guessing game. Teach them about implicit and explicit memory. Memory is like puzzle pieces that need to be put together by thinking about them. Self-reflective writing requires the right and left brain to work together and helps integration.

Teach children that emotions come and go. Feelings are temporary. Differentiate between, "I feel," and, "I am." "Feel" is a temporary state. "Am" is a trait of personality. Teach empowering language. For example, "I am stupid," versus, "This is frustrating for me right now. I know I am smart and will figure it out." Do not place judgments or labels on children because they are not doing what you want. If you do, they will become those labels. Speak only what you want to manifest.

Set behavioral intentions before an event. Plan ahead, and let kids know what is expected of them. Focus on how much they tried instead of how successful they were. Learning new skills takes time and patience. Think of how often you are not able to keep control of yourself. Their brains are still developing. Everyone makes mistakes sometimes, and they are okay. Everything is a learning experience.

Apologies are a skill to be learned. Do not force a child to apologize when they do not mean it, especially young kids, as they do not understand. There is nothing more frustrating as an adult than hearing an apology that is not genuine but used only to end a conflict. Conflicts are needed sometimes so emotions can be expressed and the person expressing them can feel heard. Start by modeling true apologies when you make mistakes. Put yourself into the other person's shoes. Show them you understand how they feel. Take responsibility for your actions. Ask what they need from you and tell them how you will work on it in the future. This sounds like a challenge, right? It sounds hard on the ego. It sure is. Do not expect your child to do something you are still working on. When you model it with them and others, they will learn, too.

As conscious parents, we want to develop balance, resilience, insight, empathy, and caring in our children. We do this by committing to listening and valuing our children, respecting, and honoring our children's feelings and needs, offering a safe space to express emotions, believing in our children, modelling behaviors, and not judging. Being a conscious parent does not mean our children are always going to be angels. Being a conscious parent means we let go of the expectation of our children having to be angels. We allow all emotions. We realize we are not responsible for our children's actions and do not have to feel shame for what they do. We are responsible for meeting our children's needs. Being a conscious parent allows us to move through all our parenting challenges peacefully. We know our children are their own beings, here on their own journey. We can do our best to be good models and love them unconditionally. We recognize we do not always know what is best for them or what experiences they should have. They have their own emotional guidance system to rely on.

One of the most beautiful things I have read on conscious parenting is from the book *Rest, Play, Grow.* Deborah MacNamara says, "Children need to rest in our care so they can play and grow." This is profound to me, even though it is so simply worded. Rest in my care. You are safe, you are accepted, you are loved, and you are appreciated. I have got this. I feel myself as Kaiden and feel the love and security I provide for him. This will allow him to find who he is as an individual, to find his own purpose for being, and to know he is safe and loved. When I give him unconditional love, through empathy, I give myself the gift, also.

Limiting Beliefs

A limiting belief is something you believe you cannot do. Henry Ford said, "Whether you think you can, or think you can't, either way you are right." In order for you to create something, you must believe it is possible. If you do not believe you can do it, you will not be able to do it. Also, in order to create something, you must not have a limiting belief around it. Abraham Hicks said something similar, "Before anything can manifest for you, there must be a vibrational compatibility between your desires and your beliefs." Either you tone down your desire, or you speed up your belief. This means you have to either make the goal smaller or increase your belief. The great thing is that a belief is just something you have thought over and over.

Most of our beliefs are not our own. They come from childhood programming. As a child, there was no filter on our subconscious. In victim consciousness, there is also no filter on the subconscious. Whatever gets put in becomes your limiting belief. A limiting belief is anything that hinders your potential to create.

This can be a religious belief, like, "God says I have to stay in my marriage even when my spouse is abusive," or, "Divorce is a sin." It can be beliefs around money, like, "Money is evil," "Money does not grow on trees," or, "You need to get a good job, work hard, and save for retirement." It could be a belief around oneself. Kids who are punished for trying things and making mistakes will have a belief that they can never do things right. You will see these people punishing themselves any time they make a mistake. They will say things to themselves, like, "You are so stupid, why can't you ever do things right?" It is like a time warp, hearing an adult in their past talking to them. Understanding this brings me huge amounts of compassion when I see people punishing themselves. It also brings understanding as to why it takes them so long to make decisions in life: they have a fear of the punishment they will inflict on themselves.

I have spent a lot of time finding my limiting beliefs and creating new empowering ones. I still have limiting beliefs stored in implicit memory in my subconscious, and they do come up from time to time. When they do, I work on them. Our spiritual journey is lifelong. We are not trying to get to a destination of perfection where happiness can finally occur. It is all about the journey of growth and finding joy in the journey.

How do we change a limiting belief to an empowering one? That is easy. We get the new one into our minds the same way the old one got into our minds: we think the thought over and over. We have all heard the saying, "If you tell a lie enough, you will start to believe it." This is because the new image rewrites the old one in the subconscious. The subconscious holds our beliefs, and it responds to repetition. We can do the exact same thing with our truths. Repeat them over and over. Your current limiting beliefs are the lies.

Another name I use for empowering beliefs is "my truth." It is not something I learned from someone else without my filter. It is something I sought out. It is something that resonates deeply inside my being. It brings me closer to source energy, to my higher self. It feels good and raises my vibration. When I stumble across these truths, the only way to describe it is revelation. Maslov calls it "peak experiences." The Buddhist term is "satori." As A Course in Miracles states, "Revelation must be experienced to understand the feeling."

I remember the first time I experienced a revelation. I was in my early twenties, still in university studying biomedicine. I was meditating on the vastness of the universe, and suddenly a thought came to me. There was a feeling of truth, almost a sense of ecstasy in knowing. Then I fell asleep. In the morning, I woke up with the feeling of revelation but could not remember what it was. I was so frustrated. Try as I might, repeating the same meditation over and over, the thought would not come. Eventually, I forgot about it. When I hired my coach Daria, and she introduced me to the Laws of Attraction, the memory came back in a meditation. The revelation I had in my twenties was: *How did someone figure out how to take a picture, and then how did it evolve into the technology of photos and motion pictures today? It all came from a thought. We can create anything from our thoughts, and our thoughts come from universal consciousness, and we all have access to it.* I know that I was not ready at that time in my life to receive that truth, so it stayed hidden until I was ready. There have been so many other revelations while reading and meditating that I have lost count. It is one of the most amazing things I have felt. That is an empowering belief.

Whenever you are working to manifest something, your desire and your belief need to be aligned. If you desire to be wealthy but have a belief that wealthy people are evil and keep poor people poor, you will have to first work on creating a new belief around wealth through repetition. In this example, it can be done by seeing all the good wealthy people do and visualizing that over and over until it sinks into the subconscious. Visualize how you would help others when you are wealthy. Whenever you are working on your "Create Your Ideal Life Meditation" from "Part Three: Spirit", you will feel discomfort if you are visualizing something that you want that conflicts with a belief you have. Write it down and work on creating a new belief through repetition. This can go for things like health, too. If you want to be healthy but truly do not believe you can be, you will want to work on the reasons why you can. Often, finding other people who have healed from something similar can help. The people who invented photographs, televisions, microwaves, lightbulbs, space crafts, and all the inventions in the world believed these impossible things were possible. They did not do it by focusing on what they did not want. They did not invent flying by focusing on falling. If they can do it, you can, too.

A Course in Miracles by Helen Schucman says, "All your misery comes from the strange belief that you are powerless. Seek not outside yourself for all your pain comes from a futile search where you insist on where it must be found. Pain is the ransom you have paid not to be freed. Your thoughts alone have caused this pain." The futile search it refers to is your search to find solutions, joy, and love outside yourself.

Exercise #24: Transform Limiting Beliefs to Empowering Beliefs: Take a piece of paper and divide it in half with a line down the middle. On the left-hand side, put "Limiting Beliefs" at the top of the page. On the right-hand side, put "Empowering Beliefs." This exercise takes self-awareness to identify the thoughts and beliefs that are causing stress. Write any limiting beliefs or stressful thoughts on the left side of the page under "Limiting Beliefs," and on the right side turn them into empowering ones. It is very important to do this as a written exercise with pen and paper. You can use pencil on the limiting beliefs so in time, you can erase them. Use your favorite color to write the empowering beliefs. When turning them around, use empowering language. Review the "Empowering Language" section for tips. When I first learned this exercise, I had books of thoughts and beliefs that were causing stress and limiting me. See the sample chart below. The section that follows goes over the process I use to create the empowering beliefs.

Limiting Belief	Empowering Belief
I always make bad decisions.	I make great decisions and learn from each and every one.
My illness cannot be cured.	I can heal. I am healing. I am so happy and grateful I have healed.
I do not do well in large groups.	I am confident. I am valuable. I speak my truth.

Limiting Beliefs Transformed to Empowering Beliefs

I cannot make money doing what I love.

If other people are able to make money doing what they love, I can, too. I am an eternal being, connected to source, and able to achieve whatever I put my mind to. Right now, I do not know how, but I can learn the tools. Empowering Beliefs: "I am learning how to make money doing what I love. I can make money doing what I love. I am easily making double my income doing what I love."

People do not want to hear what I say.

Work on confidence exercises and focus on the throat chakra in meditation. Empowering Beliefs: "I am valuable. I speak my truth, regardless of whether people are listening. I choose to have a voice. I am confident and strong."

I am too old for love.

Visualize your ideal partner. Write down a list of traits you desire in that person. Live those traits. Live as though you have found your partner. Work on self-love. Get out there and meet people online or in person. Empowering Beliefs: "I am lovable, my ideal partner is out there, and we will find each other at exactly the right time. I am open to love. I am loved."

I am not good enough.

Work on self-confidence exercises and identify where in your past this is coming from. I am an eternal being here for a human experience. God said, "I am that I am." I am that. I am that. God is also in me. I am enough. An exercise I saw done at *Train the Trainer* for this belief was to have two people on either side of you saying, "_ (Your name) _, you are enough," over and over with the audience echoing it. This lasted what felt like ten minutes. It was very powerful. If you know this is a core limiting belief, get two trusted friends who are also working on themselves to help you do this. Empowering Belief: "I am enough."

I have wasted my life and created nothing.

You are a spiritual being here for a human experience. Choose to believe that you chose to be here and learn these lessons. If you feel there is something you need to create, go create it. It is never too late. Your life has been exactly perfect to get you where you are in your consciousness today to learn tools to bring creation. You could sit in meditation for your entire life, and that would be enough. There is no wasted life, just experience. You are an eternal being. Doing Byron Katie's Work can really help when you are stuck arguing with reality. She has a way to help you see how perfect life is. Empowering Beliefs: "My life is exactly perfect the way it is. I can create now. I will live my life now."

I will be stuck with this ailment forever.

We do not know what the future will bring. We can visualize a terrible future, or we can visualize a good one. What changes is the effect on the present moment and the body. Choose to see a future where you are healthy. Feel the feeling of being healthy and achieving your goal. See "Face Your Fears" section. Empowering Beliefs: "Symptoms are a message from my body. I am determined to figure out what my body is telling me. I am healing. I am happy and grateful I am healthy."

I avoid taking risks because I am afraid of failure.

Failure does not exist unless you give up. Failure is a learning experience. With each failure, you gain new tools and are a step closer to reaching your goal. All problems are challenges that lead to growth. Life is meant to have ups and downs. Without taking risks, you will stay stuck. Empowering Belief: "I love taking risks and learning from them."

It's not Godly to want for more.

God is abundance, not lack. Money is energy. How much good could you do with more money? Look at some of the greatest spiritual teachers today and see how wealthy they are and the good they are able to do with that wealth. When you are connected to God, you are connected to the abundance of energy and are able to manifest as much as you desire. Be grateful for what you have. Focus on the exercises in the "Money Mindset" section. Work on limiting beliefs around God. Were you taught a religion and are you following it blindly? Is it really your beliefs or someone else's? Focus on learning from other spiritual teachers and reinvent your meaning of God from your truth. Empowering Beliefs: "God is abundance, I am abundance, and I am connected to abundance. I am good. I can do great things with an abundance of money."

I sound terrible when I sing and should not sing.

Most people on the planet do not sound great when they sing. We should all sing, regardless. It is okay if people do not think you sound that great, as they probably do not, either. If other people think it does not sound good, they do not have to listen. You are not responsible for how they feel. If only the great voices sang, it would be a very quiet world. This was a big one for me. I was told as a child I could not sing and should stop. That stuck with me, and I never sang in front of anyone. I did not even sing around Eric for over ten years. As I worked on my beliefs and stopped caring what others thought, I started to sing. I now sing anywhere, anytime. Empowering Beliefs: "I choose to sing the song inside me and express that joy. I love singing, and I love my voice exactly the way it is."

I am not smart enough.

Everyone has different strengths. Focus on yours. Intelligence comes in many shapes and sizes. Work on your strengths. There will be smarter and less smart people out there. Learn new skills if you feel you need to. Stop comparing, as comparison is the death of joy. You are who you are. There has never been another human being just like you. Connect with God or the universal consciousness to learn what you are capable of. Read *7 Kinds of Smart* by Thomas Armstrong. Empowering Belief: "I am a genius in my own way."

I lack money and resources.

Everyone has access to the same number of resources. Everything we could ever hope to imagine is at our fingertips. If you are lacking resources, put the effort into learning new tools. Look at time wasters and stay focused on your passions and things only you can do. Delegate and ask for help. Focus on money mindset. Learn to create abundance. Empowering Beliefs: "I am learning new tools and will manifest money. All resources come to me."

Financial security is a dream.

What we focus on, we create. Start acting and make a plan to create financial security. Focus on money mindset and self-management. Learn new tools to create abundance. You cannot create something you do not think is possible, so work on rewriting that belief. Empowering Beliefs: "I am easily attracting money to me. I am abundant. I am so happy and grateful I have achieved financial freedom."

Getting my hopes up leads to disappointments.

Hoping for something is a state of lack. Have trust and faith that you will get there at the right time. Perceived failures are really learning experiences. Be open to the universe showing alternative paths. Be grateful for what you have and where you are. Let go of attachment to end results and go for it anyway. Take action from a place of joy, passion, love, and service, not just to achieve an outcome. Empowering Beliefs:

"I love trying new things and setting big goals. All things come to me in the right time."

Life is hard, that's just the way it is.

Life is what it is. Events happen to everyone. Whether it is perceived as hard or easy depends on your self-awareness and the tools you have acquired. Work on self-confidence, and continue on your mindset journey, taking courses, attending seminars, and reading books. In time, you will feel as though you can handle anything that comes your way. If you have fears, address them. Review the "Face Your Fears" section. The way you react to an event is your point of power. The more you recognize your triggers, fears, and stressful thoughts and then learn tools to overcome them, the better your response to events will be. You are an eternal being here for a human experience. Empowering Beliefs: "I choose to make life easy. I choose to learn new tools to handle events in life. I am confident, strong, and powerful."

Others' needs are more important than mine.

If you give from lack, you will burn out and not be able to help anyone. Work on yourself first and give from abundance. When your needs are not met, you most likely will not be a pleasant person to be around and will not be able to truly meet other people's needs. It may feel like you are, but in reality, it will be coming from a place of resentment. The result will be codependency. This will hurt your relationships. Set boundaries, put yourself first, find balance, delegate, and focus on self-management and self-love. Empowering Beliefs: "My needs are the most important in my life. I am worthy, I am valuable."

I was not born into the right family.

I choose to believe that I chose my parents before coming here. I am an eternal being, and there were experiences I wanted to have. I picked my parents, as they are some of my greatest spiritual teachers. Empowering Beliefs: "I chose my family. They are my greatest spiritual teachers."

I cannot work full time and homeschool the kids.

Practice empowering language. Ask for help, reduce tasks, focus on your passions and tasks that only you can do. Delegate the rest or as much as possible. Set boundaries and say no. Work on your self-confidence and triggers. Why do I feel the need to please everyone? How did I not get approval from my parents? How does this lack of attachment affect me today? Knowing it is my child-self looking for love, how can I love myself and meet my own needs? This way I do not have to look for it from others and give away my power. What relationships in my life are toxic? Empowering Belief: "I can work full time and homeschool."

I will always avoid things because of my health.

Robert Stevens discusses the big equals in some of his talks. In math, everything you do to one side of an equation you do to the other because they equal each other. X+5 = 10, so X= 10-5. If you have a belief that "When I am healthy" equals "I will be able to do things." Then "go do things now" must equal "being healthy." No health issue should stop you from living. You have thoughts stopping you from living. If Steven Hawking can lead the field of Physics and guest star on *The Big Bang Theory*, you've got these things. Work on those thoughts. Focus on *The Work* created by Byron Katie. Ask the four questions and turn them around. Empowering Beliefs: "I choose to live now."

I always make bad decisions.

As a child, if you did something wrong, you were most likely punished. Now, as an adult when you do not make the best decision, you punish yourself instead of just taking the lack of results as new knowledge, learning from it, and moving forward. You then become afraid of failure because you punish yourself. You then second guess your gut feeling and may try a safer route. Start taking action. Stop the punishment. Take the feedback and try again. It is just new knowledge. You only fail if you give up. If it does not work, do something different. Perhaps you keep making these decisions because there is something you still need to learn. Most likely that lesson is self-confidence and self-love. Find faith that all decisions are exactly perfect because you can learn from everything. Empowering Beliefs: "I make great decisions and learn from each and every one of them."

I do not do well in large groups.

There is no such thing as doing well or not doing well. Just be, without projecting what you think people are thinking about you onto them. What they think about you is their business, and in all reality, their thoughts are on their own insecurities. They will soon forget about what you are doing. Find joy in observing people if you are uncomfortable speaking. If you want to improve your public speaking skills, join Toastmasters. The only way to improve and gain confidence is to practice until it is second nature. Empowering Beliefs: "I am confident, I am valuable, I speak my truth."

If I cannot do everything perfectly, why even bother?

Live from passion, joy, love, and service. Let go of attachment to the end result. Practice purposely not doing things well. Perfect does not exist. This is an excuse to not get started because of a fear of failure or self-inflicted judgment and punishment. Where were you punished as a child for not doing things right? Use the "Healing the Past Meditation" in "Part Three: Spirit" to help heal the trauma. Empowering Belief: "I choose to take action."

When a loved one dies, I should not be happy.

After my dog Tica died, I became numb. I felt nothing. No love, no joy, and no compassion. Nothing. I really looked inside at why I felt this way because it was not how I wanted to feel. Before Tica died, my life was full and joyous. After she died, I was unable to feel those feelings. After a lot of introspection and meditation, I realized that I had a limiting belief around death that was completely unconscious. This belief was that after the death of a loved one, I should not be happy. If you loved them, you should suffer to show how much you loved them. This belief goes deep in our society, even though consciously we may think it is silly. I knew how much I loved Tica, and Tica knew how much I loved her. I did not have to prove it to anyone or to her by being devastated. I could still feel joy, love, and happiness even though she had died. I could feel those high-vibration feelings and still miss her. I could have meltdowns and cry and be grateful, all at the same time. It hurt so much that I would never see her dog form again. It hurt for a long time. That pain, I believe, is the highest vibration of love. Each loved one's death that I have faced has turned me inward to examine the beliefs I have around death and create ones that resonate and empower me on my journey. Empowering Belief: "When a loved one dies, I embrace and express my grief, and I can still express joy and gratitude for all the good in my life."

I am a bad parent.

Immerse yourself into conscious parenting. Learn new tools to help you overcome whatever aspects of your parenting you feel are lacking. The fact that you want to try to do better means you are a good parent. Let go of the guilt and shame. It does not serve you or your kids. Remember, you were doing the best you could with the tools, knowledge, and consciousness level you were at in the past. Practice self-care. Empowering Beliefs: "I am a great parent. I am learning tools to do better. I love my kids. I love myself."

I cannot be successful without a degree.

When I first started writing this book, I wrote about twenty thousand words. They just flowed out, and it felt amazing. I was so excited to

141

share what I had learned on my journey with as many people as I possibly could. Then the fears hit. "No one will read this book because I am not a doctor," was a big one. I stopped writing and started to look into getting my Doctorate. I already have a Bachelor's in Biomedicine, so a Master's degree was my next step. I could postpone the book for those years. The thought of going back to school made me sick. Learning things I was not interested in or did not agree with, waking up early, sitting in class and doing exams all felt terrible. I had been there and done seven years of post-secondary education. I knew that was not the right path for me. When we are on course, it feels good. It is exciting. Whether you have a degree or not, people are going to judge you. The people you are meant to connect with are those who do not care if you have a degree. Look at people who do not have a degree that are ultra-successful. I also know many people who do not trust doctors and would not read a book by one. It goes either way. If people have a limiting belief that only doctors have something worthy to share, then they are missing out. That is their loss. Focus on your joy and passion and put yourself out there. Let go of attachment to results. Be of service. Empowering Beliefs: "I can be successful without a degree. I am successful."

Building Healthy Relationships

Having healthy relationships is a key to living a peaceful life. Bringing more peace to our lives is essential to healing. A common saying is that each person is responsible for fifty percent of the relationship. I personally believe that this is not the case. If we take one hundred percent responsibility and work on ourselves, our relationships change. There are four key areas I have identified that need to be focused on to build loving, peaceful relationships, and it only takes one person to do the work. These things apply to all relationships, but our relationships with our spouses are what I will focus on in this section. The people we live with, our parents, spouses, and children are the people who will bring us the most spiritual growth. We already covered relationships with children in the "Conscious Parenting" section. Here we will focus on partners, husbands, wives, boyfriends, girlfriends, spouses, or whatever name you give your significant other. This work does not happen overnight. It takes a lot of practice and there is no rushing to get to a perfect place. I have found these areas are what brought the most peace to my relationship. Eric and I have been together for fifteen years at the time of writing this book. We have been through a lot. Had it not been for the mindset work I have done, I would have a lot of resentment toward him. I would also have a lot of guilt and regret on my part for things I did or did not do. Like all mindset work, when we begin to consciously look at things, we want to remember that everyone, including ourselves, was doing and is doing the best they can with the tools, skills, knowledge, and level of consciousness they are at. It is a learning process. The areas of importance are unconditional love, recognizing the ego, recognizing and addressing triggers, and healthy communication.

The first area that has really helped my relationship is expressing unconditional love. For a long time in my relationship, before I started my mindset journey and became conscious of my own behaviors, when Eric and I had an argument, my thoughts were of leaving him. Often, our fights would end up with me threatening to leave. I would think of how much better it could be if I had another man that was different. The grass is always greener on the other side. Often, he would say, "Well if you are not happy, there is the door." Obviously, I never left despite that, but since doing the mindset work, I realized the grass is not greener on the other side. More often than not, when someone leaves a dysfunctional relationship, they attract the same type of person again. The lesson repeats itself until the lesson is learned. Once the lesson is learned, there is rarely a reason to leave as the issues go away. Your triggers, reactions, and lack of communication are what cause the arguing and fighting.

All anyone truly wants is to be loved unconditionally. Most parents love their children unconditionally and most kids, though they may not get along with their parents, also love their parents unconditionally. When I realized this in my mindset work while learning about the needs of a child, I decided to love Eric unconditionally. This was a decision to not ever threaten to leave again and to move to love even after arguments. I went back and explored every single thing about which I held any resentment toward him and took responsibility for it. I wrote down each one and then went back and asked myself, "How could I have responded differently and changed the situation had I been more confident in myself?" I also saw in each situation how we were doing the best we could and how that situation contributed to where I am today. I grew from each situation. I have found that when I hold any resentment toward him for anything, even something small, it affects my mood. Whenever we have an argument or I feel upset with him, I move back to unconditional love as soon as possible. Even if I have not worked through it by the end of day, I let him know how much I love him regardless.

Exercise #25: Moving Past Resentments: Write a list of anything for which you resent your partner. These offenses can be big or small. Ask yourself how you created or allowed the situation. How could you have changed the situation had you been more confident? What could you have done differently? How did you not express yourself? What did you learn from the situation? How did it make you a better person? If there is anything that needs to be expressed, express it.

A tool that helps me move back to unconditional love is to question any thought I have about him. For example, if I think, "He is being so lazy," I ask myself, "Is it true?" Then I find proof he is not lazy. If I feel he is not doing enough, I ask myself, "Is it true?" and immediately I will remember things that he does which illustrates otherwise. I also ask myself how I feel when I believe this story. Our thoughts become stories that are often fictional. When we stop believing the story and recognize how it is not true, we change our lives. This technique is from Byron Katie's *The Work*. By questioning the judgment I have about him, I recognize they are not true. This allows me to shift from what I do not like to what I do like. When I am judging him or feeling resentment, this also helps me to shift focus on how I also do the same things. People are always a mirror for something you either do yourself or for where you need to be more like them. Other tools to shift back to unconditional love include: recognizing how my ego is trying to make him wrong, focusing on his good qualities, and thinking about what I am grateful for and appreciate about him.

There are three types of love: human, spiritual, and divine love. Most human love tends to be based on the premise, "I love you as long as you are pleasing me. When you are not pleasing me, I do not love you and can have no problem leaving you." Spiritual love is unconditional love. It is the love we most often see between mother and child, and sometimes between father and child. It can also be the deep love a child has for their parents when attachment is secure. It does not waiver no matter how the person is behaving. Divine love is unconditional love for all beings, seeing everyone as parts of God or universal consciousness. It is the love of great spiritual teachers. Everyone wants to feel unconditionally loved. Divine love and spiritual love come from your spirit; human love comes from the ego. When we give unconditional love to someone, when we see them as a spiritual being, when we let go of all judgments on them and their past and love them exactly as they are, we give ourselves unconditional love as well. We can feel the acceptance, love, approval, and understanding they are receiving, and we experience it ourselves.

The second area that has really helped me have a healthy relationship is recognizing the ego. In relationships, the ego says, "I want to be right. I want to win. I want you to make me happy. I want you to be more like me. You should do this." The first step is to become conscious of your ego taking over and feeling one of the above. This takes a lot of work to happen in the moment. Usually, it happens in the reflection stage, where you reflect on your feelings of anger, resentment, and frustration after an argument. Ask yourself, "Is this my ego talking? Am I trying to make the other person wrong? Am I wanting them to make me happy or be more like me?" From there, you can tell yourself how no one likes to be made wrong. When you make someone wrong, you are trying to get them to feel guilty. It is a form of manipulation. Tell yourself also that there is no right or wrong. There is only perception. Ask yourself,

"How am I taking this too seriously? Is this really important? Am I overreacting?" Remember the quote from *A Course in Miracles*, "I can choose peace rather than this." It also states that peace is the ego's greatest enemy. As I am writing this, I just did this tonight. I actually laughed at the synchronicity, knowing I was coming to read over this section and make edits. Kaiden fell asleep on me while Eric and I watched our show together. Before bed, Kaiden had dipped the remote for the TV into a glass of water and it was not working that well. He had just fallen asleep as the show ended. Eric had muted the TV and then tried to turn it off. He started to talk, asking me where the other remote was, and Kaiden woke up; he did not just wake up a bit, he was wide awake. It then took me another hour to get him back to sleep. While Kaiden ran room to room, I laid in bed and reflected on what I was feeling. I immediately saw my ego trying to make Eric wrong. I recognized that it really did not matter that Kaiden had woken up, and that Eric was not purposely trying to wake him up, either.

Always look at the situation from the other person's perspective. I became present and found joy in Kaiden's joy as he ran in and out of Eric's room with glee. Instead of making Eric wrong, I learned from it and will make reminders before we watch the show for both of us not to start talking when the volume is off. Though I did not say to him that he was wrong, he could sense it from the frustration in my tone. He would have felt I was blaming him, which I did until I went to reflect on what had happened. After I edited this section, I went to apologize. Apologies are hard for the ego. Apologizing does not mean feeling guilty and beating yourself up. It is all about the learning process.

It is a good time to mention again that mindset training is not about not feeling emotions or suppressing them. I allowed myself to feel frustrated that Kaiden woke up. I just did not stay there long. It is not wrong to feel lower-vibration emotions for long periods, either. It is not wrong to have extreme anger or hate, or to react strongly, but it does not feel good. It is stressful to the body. I prefer to feel peace and joy. Though we cannot feel that all the time, there are many tools to move out of those states if you also desire to feel peace and joy.

The process of reflecting on my thoughts and moving past the resentment took about ten minutes. Before mindset work, I would hold in each resentment, replaying it over and over in my head, unable to get past why he was wrong and what he should be doing. When the resentments built up and caused too much tension, I would explode them all out in a fiery rage of yelling and tears. When I started mindset work, the reflection process could take up to a week or longer. That time has gradually reduced, and now I often can reflect in the moment. If not, then it happens soon after. I allow myself to feel the emotion, then reflect and express. I do not push it away or let it build up for later. I learn from it, set a boundary for next time, and try to express it in a way that does not trigger the other person.

It is worth mentioning that though I believe working on oneself can create a healthy relationship, I would not tolerate any physical abuse. There are many reasons why people stay in abusive relationships, and that is beyond the scope of this book. If you are experiencing physical abuse, please seek professional help.

Recall in the "Conscious Parenting" section, when children have a tantrum or strong emotions, there is no point in trying to reason with them while they are in that state. The lower, primitive brain has taken over, and reasoning will not happen. Calmness has to occur for self-reflection to take place. This happens in adults, also. If you find yourself in a disagreement that has escalated into yelling and extreme anger, it is best to leave the situation. State that you will only speak in calm, respectful voices. The ego will try to be right and want you to respond. When both parties are calm, that is the time to work on the issue.

The ego wants everyone else to be like you and change to make you happy. This is not going to happen, ever. The world is full of dichotomies and opposites to show you what you want and what you do not want. When we recognize happiness comes from within and no one else can make us happy, we stop expecting other people to do it for us.

Exercise #26: Should List: You may feel that your partner should be doing things differently. Write a list of all the shoulds that your partner, or anyone else in your life, should be doing. For example, "My partner should exercise more. My partner should spend more time with the kids. My partner should be tidier. My partner should eat better. My partner should not get so angry all the time." Now cross out "my partner" and put "I." "I should …" Do the work on yourself, and lead from example.

The third key to a healthy relationship is to recognize your triggers and work on yourself. We discussed triggers in depth in the "Conscious Parenting" section. A good way to tell you are triggered is that you react in a way that is more intense than the situation warrants. You are returning to something from your past, most likely from your childhood. When you notice these more-intense-than-expected reactions, take some time to reflect. When you ask your subconscious a question, it usually answers. Ask yourself, "Where in my past has this happened before? Is there a limiting belief here?" Use the "Healing the Past Meditation" in "Part Three: Spirit" to help you heal from past emotional trauma. A great exercise is to ask your partner what skills they think you should work on. Ask them, "What does our relationship need in order to be better for you? What are areas I can work on that you feel would help me grow?" Usually, if we can tame our egos and listen, our partners know us well enough to tell us exactly where we need to do some work.

Exercise #27: Get Clear on Who You Want to Be: What kind of person have I been? Is there an emotion I struggle with every day? This could be anger, frustration, hate, resentment, etc. How would my friends and family describe me? Do I hide how I truly feel? What is something I want to change about myself? Who do I admire? What qualities do I admire about them? What would it take to think like them? What can I practice daily to create these qualities in myself?

Jealousy and insecurity in relationships are an indication the person feeling those emotions needs to do work on their confidence. Trust comes from a confidence in yourself and in the universe. There is no way you can control another person's behavior. That is codependency. No amount of controlling another person's behavior by knowing where they are or what they are doing will stop someone from cheating. It is directly the opposite. Those people feeling controlled and untrusted are more likely to seek love elsewhere. Jealousy is a big turn off for most people. I used to be so jealous and worried Eric would cheat on me. He is a musician and would be off playing out of town for lots of people, including lots of women. Most of them would drink and then go off to a hotel room. My thoughts would see him with other women. It was never about him. It took a lot of growth to realize that if he cheated on me, that is on his karma, not mine. My focus needs to be on my confidence and not needing him to be faithful in order for me to be happy.

Neurotransmitter imbalance can lead to more obsessive-compulsive thoughts, usually pointing to low serotonin. Increasing serotonin can help significantly with the thoughts, but the underlying self-confidence needs to be addressed. It is coming to a place where if your spouse cheated on you, you would be okay. You could either forgive them or move on without them. After having a child and making a firm commitment to love Eric unconditionally, now if he cheated, I really would be okay with it. Our love and connection are very deep, and I know it would have just been sex. That is where I am now. Five years ago, I was not at this place. At that time, I needed him to make me happy. Now, I do not need him to make me happy. I am happy. Insecurity says, "I need you to need me. I need you to want me. If you do not, I will not be okay." Love says, "I want you to be happy. If your happiness is with another person, I will be okay."

The fourth key in creating a healthy relationship is to learn healthy communication. As discussed in the "Conscious Parenting" section, most of us never learned how to properly communicate. Many parents punished any expressed emotions as misbehavior, and most parents do not model healthy communication. That model became you. It is not too late to learn how to do the opposite. Emotions are not bad. When you are feeling any lower-vibration emotion, allow it. Feel it. Do not fight against it. Name what you are feeling. See where you feel it in your body. Observe it with nonjudgment. Soothe yourself as you would a child that has just hurt themselves. Show empathy and compassion to yourself. Seek a safe person to express your emotions to, if needed.

Someone who understands how to show empathy. Allow yourself to return to calm. A meditation can help with this. When you are calm, reflect on your thoughts. Recognize your ego and triggers, see the other person's point of view, and do the work on your thoughts. When the other person is calm, express how you feel using "I" statements. "I feel _____," versus, "You made me feel _____."

Most people fall under one of two types of emotional expression: those who immediately express how they feel about you and the situation, and those who bottle things up, use the silent treatment, and seem calm while they are seething. The former will often swear and yell. The latter may deprive you of their love and affection, then eventually explode. Eric is definitely the first type, and I am definitely the second, though I have done significant work on it. When I started to do mindset work, I realized how we were both being triggered. When we had a conflict, I would cry, and he would yell. In recognizing I was triggered, I would stop and gather myself until I could speak calmly without using the tears as a weapon. They were not a conscious weapon but nonetheless, they were a way to try to make him feel guilty. I also set a non-negotiable boundary of not being yelled at. Since then, I say, "We are both upset and need some time to calm down. We can discuss this when we can both speak to each other calmly." Then, I leave the room. If you are so mad that you need to yell, do not express your emotion at someone. Leave the room, go outside, and let it out. Punch a punching bag. Get it all out. Then, reflect on the emotions. After that, express how you feel safely to the other person.

Not expressing the emotions while seething inside is swallowing poison and expecting the other person to die. Overall, the person who expresses their frustration will be able to move on, whereas the person who does not will replay it over and over in their mind. The person who holds it in is often afraid of the angry outburst from the other person. This is why healthy communication is so important to develop. A healthy medium is needed between the two types of expression. The person who immediately blows up needs to work on returning to calm and reflection. The person who bottles things in needs to work on expression and moving to expression more quickly. At the end of the day, you cannot make someone address their triggers or want to work on self-growth. They are on their own journey and will come to it when they are ready. All you can do is work on yourself and lead by example.

Face Your Fears

Fear and desire felt together equal courage. Every situation we find ourselves in has a cost and a benefit; a pro and a con. The reason we stay stuck in situations we do not like is because we do not want to face a fear. We may not like the situation we are in, but we do not want to risk facing the fear. It is safer to stay where we are because it is comfortable. Everything you desire is going to be outside of your comfort zone. Growth will require you to face your fears. If the thing you desired was inside your comfort zone, you would have done it already. The opposite of love is not hate. It is fear. Fear can be big or small.

In today's world, most of our fears are not going to physically harm us. Fear of being judged, fear of failing, fear of success, fear of being disliked, fear of confrontation: none of these will cause us physical harm. Fears can be of situations, places, creatures, or the paranormal. Common fears are dying, public speaking, spiders, and dentists. Remember that the brain is unable to tell the difference between a thought and a real event. Fear is imagining what you do not want to happen, which then causes a cortisol response in the body. Review the "Understanding the Cortisol Response" section to review how the stress response affects our bodies. The stress response can range from mild to debilitating.

Fear is negative goal setting. Though we know we can choose our thoughts, when it comes to intense fear, especially when it is a common pattern for the person, it can be difficult to refocus on what we want due to lack of prefrontal integration. I want to share some tools that have helped me work through and overcome my fears.

Reaction planning and mental rehearsal are tools where you take some time to imagine how you would like an event to go. You play out the situation beforehand. For example, if you have a fear of confrontation, and you know you will be put into an uncomfortable situation that may cause anxiety, you can take the time to decide what you want to say and imagine how the person will respond. You can see yourself being confident and prepared, and the situation being resolved. If you are going to give a speech, you can visualize yourself giving it over and over until you feel comfortable. Go into detail and see the before and after. Feel yourself being confident and feel the relief and feeling of accomplishment after it is finished. If you are afraid of dentists, visualize going to the office, taking deep breaths, being calm during your procedure and then your sense of relief at the end of the visit.

Often, we start to imagine terrible things happening and do not even notice we are doing it. The thought pattern takes over, and the next thing we know, we are in full-blown anxiety even though we are perfectly safe. An exercise I like to use to pop me out of fear and into the present is to ask myself, "Right now, am I safe?" The answer is almost always yes. If you truly are not safe at the time, please seek help. If in the present moment you are safe, say to yourself, "I scare myself by imagining…" Then ask yourself, "If I weren't afraid, what would I do?" This works really well for ego-related fears: fear of being judged, fear of failure, and fear of success.

Another tool to use when trying to face a fear is to break things down into small steps. If you are afraid of public speaking, start by talking in front of a mirror, graduate to speaking in front of an intimate group, and then find a place to talk in front of a small group. As you gain confidence, you can schedule speaking engagements with a larger audience. Each small fear you face will bring confidence. When kids learn to jump into water, they do not go straight to the high dive. They make gradual approximations toward the desired goal. First jumping from the edge, then from the swimmer's block, then from the small dive, and eventually from the higher ones.

For more serious fears, I go through an exercise I developed called "worst-case, best-case, present." One of the best ways to discover your fears and limiting beliefs is to imagine what you are afraid of, from the beginning to the end. See it from the third person point of view and ask yourself, "And then what happens? And then what happens?" It is like you are watching a movie of your fear instead of being the actor in it.

For example, I had a client who was afraid to go out because she would get dizzy. I had her imagine herself going out and getting dizzy. She saw herself going to the store. I asked her, "And then what happens?"

She said, "I start to feel dizzy, and I get scared that I am going to pass out."

"And then what happens?"

"I fall over."

"And then what happens?"

"People help me."

"And then what happens?"

"Someone calls an ambulance."

"And then what happens?"

"I get taken to the hospital, and they do tests."

"And then what happens?"

"Then my husband comes to get me."

When we further analyzed it, her fears were of what other people would think of her if she passed out, of being seen as vulnerable, and of asking for help. All of her fears were ones that could be addressed. We went deeper by asking, "What will the people really think?"

She replied, "They will just want to help. They will feel concern, and some may not even care. At the end of the day, they will all go back to their lives, and it will not be a big deal for them."

"Where does your fear of asking for help originate?"

"When I was a child, any time I would ask for help, my mother would get mad at me. She was so busy, and I was interrupting her. She would tell me I was being a baby and could do it myself." Bingo.

It is important to face the fears in your mind so you can identify the root cause of the fear. Then you can create an empowering belief around those fears. When you know the fear is coming from your child-self, it is easier to face it because you know you are not a child anymore. In the above example, new beliefs would be, "It is okay to ask for help. People truly want to help. It is healthy to show my emotions and vulnerability. It is okay to talk about my health." These would be important to repeat on a daily basis. When the fears are identified, they can be broken down. In this example, starting to show vulnerability to friends and family by talking about her health issues was a first step. Then she started going with her husband to church, where she could discuss her health issues and fears in a safe place. It was not long before she was able to go out again by herself, knowing if she did pass out, she would be okay.

I often get resistance to going into the worst-case scenario after people have learned about the Laws of Attraction. They ask, "Won't it cause me to create what I do not want because I am thinking about it?" The Laws of Attraction do not work like that. Negative thoughts are much less powerful than positive ones. It takes thinking about something for a long time for most people to create it. The point of attraction is in the feeling. The exercise is meant to allow you to get to the root cause of the fear and limiting belief so you can work through it and then face the fear. This is much better than ignoring the fear or staying in a constant place of anxiety. This is bringing consciousness and self-awareness to it. It brings light and sends away the darkness. After the worst-case scenario is done and the fears and limiting beliefs are processed, move to the next phase of the exercise.

The first time you do this exercise, it takes longer because you are identifying your fears, creating new affirmations, and making action steps. The fears will still pop into your mind. When that happens, you are able to quickly go through the worst-case scenarios, use your affirmations, and realize that in the end, you are okay. After you do the worst-case scenario, move to the best-case scenario. For the second part of the exercise, imagine how you want the event to go. For the above example, she would see herself going out and feeling great. If the feeling of dizziness comes on, she sits down and regroups herself. Perhaps she asks for help. She sees herself discussing her fears and her dizziness with people. She comes home and feels a sense of accomplishment and connection.

The third part of the exercise is to move into presence. Immerse yourself in a task. It can be a breathing exercise or something as simple as doing the dishes. Feel the water and smell the soap. The process is repeated until the anxiety dissipates. Doing one of the meditations from "Part Three: Spirit" is a great way to come into presence.

While working on this section, I used this technique to help me process a fear. Kaiden hit his tooth a couple months ago. We were hoping the tooth would recover, but sadly it did not. In order to save the tooth, Kaiden would have to be put under anesthesia and have his tooth repaired. I have done a lot of work on my fear around dentists, and I can now fall asleep during dental work with my meditation exercises. Though I have also done a lot of work around my fear of Kaiden dying, it will always be there. The beliefs I have put in place around death have allowed me to not be controlled by the fear. When I was talking to the dentist, my mind immediately went to, "What if he dies when they put him under anesthesia?" I asked myself how those thoughts would help the situation. How would sitting here terrified help him get through it? I have gone to the worst-case scenario and have walked myself through that before. I affirm my belief that we are all here for exactly the right amount of time. We are all eternal beings here to learn, teach, and experience. I then moved to best-case scenario. I told myself that Kaiden has great phase one detoxification pathways, as Eric and I do. His phase two detoxification is supported, and phase three should be functioning well, as he has had minimal toxin exposure in his life. I saw myself calmly rocking him the night before, as he would not be able to nurse for hours prior. I saw myself getting up and quickly heading out the door to his appointment that morning, as he would not be able to eat. He loves car rides.

I saw him content. I saw him quickly falling asleep with the mask. I saw myself there for him when he would wake up. I saw him eating and happy afterward, as I knew that I felt fine after being put under. Then, I immersed myself in a task. I was at the barn when the dentist called. After talking to the dentist, I felt the fear. I expressed it. I cried. I walked myself through the best-case scenario, and then I got on my horse and trotted off bareback. I felt my weight shift with each of Vala's hoof falls, as I breathed in and out. With each exhale, my tension left me, went into Vala, and then out through each thunder of her hooves hitting the ground. My tension eased. Because I had done so much work on my beliefs around death, I did not have to go to the worst-case scenario often. When the thoughts of the dentist came, I would go to best-case, see it to completion, see the outcome I desired, and then return to a present activity. Kaiden's dentist appointment went well. He has a nice white tooth. There was crying from both of us, but we overcame the challenge and are stronger from it.

Guilt and Resentment

To shift into a high vibration and to heal, it is important to address any guilt and resentment you are holding. Guilt only serves us in the present moment. Thinking, "I will not hurt that person because I do not want to feel guilty," prevents you from acting. After an event has occurred, we feel guilty as a form of punishment. We feel guilty because we have been taught that good people feel guilty when they do something wrong. They show remorse. Bad people do not. In reality, if a person does not feel guilty after hurting someone, then they are not at a level of consciousness to be aware of what they did. When you look back at your past, you look at yourself with your current knowledge, skills, and consciousness level. You were not the same person then, and it is not fair to yourself to hold your past self to your current self's standards. Had you known what you know now, you would have chosen a different response. No amount of punishing yourself is going to change a past event. When we take responsibility for our lives, we realize that everyone, including ourselves, was doing and is doing the best they can with the tools, knowledge, and skills they have at the time. We do not brush guilt under the rug with the blanket statement of, "I was doing the best I could." Allow yourself to feel the guilt, learn from it, decide what you would do differently, and apologize. Review true apologies in the "Conscious Parenting" section. You can also use the "Heal Your Past Meditation" in "Part Three: Spirit" to help. Forgive yourself, learn from the past, and grow. Guilt allows you to maintain a belief that you are good. When you realize that at the core of your being, you are good and have always tried to be good, forgiveness comes. The same goes for everyone else. We all want to be good. We all want to be loved. There is no need to punish yourself for the rest of your life for something that happened in the past.

There is a big difference between shame and guilt. Guilt says, "My behavior was bad," while shame says, "I am bad." Both can be used to fuel self-growth. For shame, we want to rewrite our beliefs about ourselves. See the "Limiting Beliefs" section for tools to do this. I also love Brene Brown's talks and books on shame and vulnerability. For guilt, we need to create a new belief around the event that serves us.

A common reason people feel guilty is because they were not there when a loved one died. For example, my dog Tica died while I was away for Jack Canfield's training. "A good dog mom is there when her dog dies," was creating guilt for me. Since my belief did not match reality, I felt guilty. I felt I was a bad dog mom. By amending the belief, the guilt goes away. I created a new belief that had I known she was going to die, I would have been there for her. I did not know she was going to die. No amount of guilt will bring her back. I also created the belief that she wanted me to go so she could move on. Had I been there, I may have been able to prevent it. I had been keeping her alive for that past year. I believe she was ready. I also look back and ask myself if I am a good dog mom. The answer is yes. Knowing I am good at the core of my being allows me to let go of the guilt.

Exercise #28: Letting Go of Guilt: To summarize the steps above, first think of something that makes you feel guilty. Determine the belief you created during this event. Amend the belief, knowing you were doing the best you could with your skills, knowledge, and consciousness level during that time. Create new beliefs around the event and get in touch with your inner goodness. Decide what you would do differently in the future if it happened again. Reflect on what you learned from the situation. If needed, give a true apology.

Resentment is resending anger, hate, and frustration over and over after the initial event that hurt you is over. Healing from it is similar to guilt, as we recognize the other person was doing the best they could with the tools, knowledge, and skills they had. Taking responsibility for how you created or allowed the event that made you feel resentment is also needed. When we take responsibility for our lives, the resentment disappears, and forgiveness becomes unnecessary.

Money Mindset

Money is energy; it is infinite, unlimited, and there is an abundance for everyone. When I first started learning about mindset training, I was focused on building my business and making money. I had reached my health goals, so my focus turned to creating wealth. I had a very poor money mindset. *Money does not grow on trees. Rich people are evil. Money corrupts people. Work hard to retire.* These were some of the beliefs I had around money. I also did not value myself or my knowledge. I felt guilty accepting money from people and felt I should work for very little or for free. When I started working through my limiting beliefs with my coach, the first sentence of this section became my mantra. I now truly believe that money is energy, and there is an abundance for everyone. I went from working hard and making little money to working smart and making lots. Anyone can do it. It just takes a massive paradigm shift. I am very grateful to my coach Daria Zest for helping me make that shift. I have saved the limiting beliefs about money for this section and will share tools to make the shift from a poor mindset to a wealth consciousness.

Creating affirmations around money to replace limiting beliefs is a valuable tool in shifting to wealth consciousness. Here are some empowering beliefs that have helped me:

- ☐ Money is coming to me effortlessly from multiple sources every day.
- ☐ There is an unlimited supply of money.
- ☐ I am open to receiving.
- ☐ I give myself permission to be wealthy.
- ☐ I am worthy of making more money.
- ☐ I love money.

- ☐ I use money to better my life and the lives of others.
- ☐ I am aligned with the energy of abundance.
- ☐ My finances improve every day.
- ☐ Money is the root of joy and comfort.
- ☐ Money and spirituality can co-exist in harmony.
- ☐ I easily handle large sums of money.
- ☐ Gratitude is key in attracting abundance.
- ☐ Money helps to find freedom, generosity, and compassion.

Exercise #29: Identify Your Beliefs Around Money:

- ☐ What beliefs around money do you have?
- ☐ What beliefs about money have you inherited from your parents?
- ☐ What doubts and fears do you have about yourself and money?
- ☐ What judgments do you have around people who are wealthy?
- ☐ How are you being cheap with yourself?
- ☐ How will you stop being cheap with yourself?
- ☐ What do you think might stop you from making consistent money?
- ☐ What do you desire to do but keep yourself from doing because of fear of being judged by others?
- ☐ Whose approval are you trying to get?
- ☐ Who are you afraid will judge you?
- ☐ Let go of judgment. What do you need to do?
- ☐ What money beliefs do you choose to eliminate?
- ☐ What money beliefs do you consciously choose? (You can use the list above.)
- ☐ What does it feel and look like to you to be wealthy?
- ☐ What meaning does money have for you? (Examples: freedom, traveling, comfort, security, etc.)

Exercise #30: Living from Abundance: Take your yearly income, and in your head turn it into your monthly income. If you make $60k a year, visualize making $60k per month. How does it feel making your yearly income in a month?

Fill out the information below imagining that your yearly income became your monthly income.

- ☐ The decisions I make today are:
- ☐ My life looks like:
- ☐ I choose to:
- ☐ I am purchasing:
- ☐ I am traveling to:
- ☐ I am delegating the following tasks to:
- ☐ I am prioritizing my self-care by:

Exercise #31: Money Always Needs a Purpose: Write down how much money you need to spend on what items and the purpose. Do not rationalize it, as the whole point is in letting yourself dream bigger than your mind normally does.

- ☐ What amount of money do you need to spend?
- ☐ For what purpose do you need it?
- ☐ Why do you fear you will not receive this money?
- ☐ Why do you think you do not deserve this money?

Change your perspective.

- ☐ Why do you know you will receive this money?
- ☐ Why do you know you do deserve this money?
- ☐ What do you need to change in yourself to be the person with that level of wealth?

Exercise #32: Get Clear on Your Passion: The key to making money is to be of service by either providing an amazing service that helps people or creating a product that helps people. This must be a product or service you love, value, and believe in. Get in touch with your passion and purpose, what you are good at, and the knowledge you have that will allow you to be of service. The below questions will dig into your subconscious and allow you to get in touch with your true self.

- [ ] What did you love to do as a child?
- [ ] What comes easily and naturally to you?
- [ ] What would you do for free every day just because you love it?
- [ ] What would be the most joyful way for you to make money?
- [ ] If there were no consequences or limitations, what would you do now? And how would you do it?
- [ ] Look for a common thread in all of your above answers. What is your *why* in life?
- [ ] If you had millions of dollars and did not need to work to make money, what would you do?
- [ ] Look at the above answers. What business, service, or product could you create?

Exercise #33: Get Clear on Your Vision: Getting clear and focusing on our visions helps attract the means to create the visions. Let go of the how and focus on the end result. See it as though it is already here. Be open and allow the path to unfold as you take steps in the direction of your vision. Using the product, service, or business above, answer the following questions.

- [ ] How do you desire your career/business to feel?
- [ ] What type of clients do you desire?
- [ ] How much time do you desire to work in your business?
- [ ] What type of business do you desire to grow or work for (small team up to ten people, mid-size company up to fifty people, corporation, etc.)?
- [ ] Describe below, in detail, how your ideal workday would look. Be very specific. Details matter. Infuse your core values, how your business makes you feel, what kind of clients you are working with, who is on your team, where you are located, how many hours you work, and how your overall lifestyle looks.
- [ ] What is your monthly financial goal?
- [ ] What are the results your clients can expect from working with you? Or what results will your product give to people? Be specific.

Exercise #34: Money Opportunities: Think about opportunities money gives you in life and how money makes you a better person. For example, money makes me kinder because I can help others more when I have money. I only listed five, but you can list as many as you want. I did the first one for you.

1. I love money because it gives me the freedom to travel.

2.

3.

4.

5.

Exercise #35: Gratitude: A key to attracting money into your life is to shift out of lack. Focus on gratitude for what you do have instead of thinking about what you do not have. Write a list of everything for which you are grateful. Whenever you find your vibration lowering, go over your list and feel the gratitude.

Shifting out of lack helps create wealth consciousness. A great way to do this is to act as if you already have money. Feel as you would if you were wealthy. Watch where you count points or always look for deals. This creates a state of lack. Competition is also a state of lack. It is saying there is not enough to go around. Trust that there is enough for everyone. Wish success for everyone.

Another way to shift the vibration is to give money away. Donating a percent of your income to charities that are meaningful to you brings abundance back to you. Money is energy, and it needs to flow. When it flows out, it comes back. Giving shows you trust that you will receive it back. Giving is the ultimate way to move out of lack. It is such a great feeling to give to others, especially anonymously.

There are many great books and audio programs on wealth consciousness. Some of my favorites are:

- *Think and Grow Rich* by Napoleon Hill.
- *The Science of Getting Rich* by Wallace D. Wattles.
- *The Secret to Attracting Money* by Joe Vitale.
- *Your Creative Soul* by Caroline Myss and Sandra Joseph.
- *Money and The Laws of Attraction* by Esther Hicks.
- *It's Not About the Money* by Bob Proctor.
- *The Big Leap* by Gay Hendricks.

Self-Sabotage and the Upper Limit Principle

Often when we set a goal, we have to face fears in order to reach it. Most things we are afraid of are not actually going to hurt us, such as asking for help, applying for a new job, or speaking in front of a large audience. Our bodies do not know the difference between a real threat and an imagined threat. When we have to move out of our comfort zones and face fear, the subconscious mind will try to keep us safe by preventing us from having to face the fear. A good example was a client who was facing a fear of travelling on her own. Right before she had to face the fear, she got sick with a bad flu. She was not able to go on the trip. Often, right before we have to face a fear, we end up getting injured or sick. Another example is how on the day of a presentation, the car breaks down. These little things that may seem like a coincidence really are the subconscious and the Laws of Attraction at work. Self-sabotage is unconscious. It happens. Expect it. Plan for it. Face the fear anyway. Something that helps me is to say to my fear, "Thank you for trying to keep me safe. You are welcome to come along for the ride, but you are not allowed to drive." While I was writing this book, often when I started with a new section, self-sabotage would kick in. For example, the day I was starting the "Building Healthy Relationships" section, Eric and I had a huge argument. My ego would say, "How can you write a section on relationships when you just had this conflict? Best to give up now and not write the book." Fear of being judged and fear of failing came back full force. Instead of giving in, I used the principles I wrote about, and we worked through the conflict very quickly. I used the conflict to fuel me instead of stopping me, as it showed how well the principles work.

Upper limit principle and self-sabotage go hand in hand. Our upper limit is a goal that will put us to our perceived next level. For example, if you usually make around $10k a month and have a goal to reach $15k but just never seem to make it, then $15k becomes your upper limit. It could also be an amount of money in your bank account. You get so close to saving $100k, but every time you are about to make it over that amount, something happens: your car breaks down, you need dental work, or your furnace needs to be replaced. Your upper limit is $100k. Whenever we set a goal that seems too big and we are about to reach it, something will happen to prevent the goal from being reached. I have found just bringing awareness to the fact that I am stuck in an upper limit principle is enough to help me break through it. I visualize there being a ceiling over me. It is my upper limit. It is my comfort zone. My goal is on the other side. I visualize myself as Superwoman, one fist raised in the air, flying straight through the ceiling, and shattering it into a thousand pieces. I also like to create new affirmations around the goal. From the above examples, affirmations would sound like, "I am easily making twenty thousand every month." "I am so happy and grateful I have a hundred and ten thousand in my account." I also feel the accomplishment and hear myself telling Eric, "I broke through my ceiling!"

Turning Inward

When healing from illness, it is imperative to get the body to a peaceful state. Healing does not occur when the body is stressed, depressed, anxious, or feeling any lower-vibration emotions on a regular basis. It is totally normal and healthy to feel all of those emotions. We just do not want to get stuck there and have it become our attraction point. "Part Two: Mind" has been all about learning how our thoughts affect our bodies and that we have the power to choose our thoughts. The tools presented were to help you learn to shift your vibration to a higher one that allows healing to occur. In order to do this, you have to make the time available for yourself. We looked at self-management and how to fit in self-care, the most important of self-care being mindset training. We also took a look at your stressors and time wasters, and freed up time for you.

Then, you learned how to upgrade to empowering language and how to help protect your energy and build confidence. I shared the tools to help you create your ideal life. I also explained how to get clear on what you want and use goal setting and affirmations to motivate you to take action toward your goals.

An introduction to conscious parenting helped you see where your limiting beliefs came from and what shaped you to be who you are today. The tools in that section will help bring peace to your relationships with the children in your life. After seeing where your limiting beliefs originated, you were able to dive deep into identifying your limiting beliefs and turning them into empowering ones.

From there, we discussed tools to help create happy, healthy relationships. Most of our stress in life comes from our relationship problems. Finding peace here is vital to healing. We discussed how to bring empathy into your relationships without a drain on energy, facing your fears that are holding you back from reaching your goals, and working through guilt and resentment to free the burden on your soul. We finished off with the always exciting work on money mindset, which taught you how to use your newfound power to create wealth in your life.

Now we are moving to "Part Three: Spirit," where we will work on getting in touch with your passion and purpose. I will share with you an easy meditation practice to help you go further into yourself on your spiritual journey.

PART THREE

SPIRIT

Passion and Purpose

We are all born with passion inside of us. We are here to create, experience, learn, teach, expand, and grow. Our passions and purposes fuel our souls. Too often, limiting beliefs keep us from pursuing our passions and purposes. Limiting beliefs include statements like, "I cannot make this a career; it will not make any money. I need to work hard and save for retirement, then I can enjoy life," and, "It is my responsibility to pay for my kids to go to school. Their happiness is more important than my own." We get caught up in the rat race, doing what other people think is best for us, and living with "shoulds." When we get stuck in a dead-end job that causes stress and is not enjoyable, the soul is deprived of its fuel. That leads to depression and anxiety. Society tells us to push through, there is something wrong with you, and there is a pill to help. In truth, it is an existential crisis. Our emotions are there to tell us when we are on or off course. High-vibration emotions tell you that you are on course. Low-vibration emotions tell you that you are off course. Turning off those emotions with a medication is like turning off your car's check-engine light without figuring out why it came on in the first place. Your soul is your connection to source energy. This energy is limitless, and you are tapped into it all the time if you open yourself up to it. If you ignore the messages from your higher self, you will feel increasingly worse.

Meditation helps you get in touch with your higher self. It helps you find your passion and purpose. Your passion is anything that brings you joy. You can tell you have found it when you are excited. Passions and purposes change throughout life, and you may have more than one. The key is to follow your joy. The word "enthusiasm" has the root *enthous*, meaning "possessed by a God, inspired." When you feel enthusiasm, you know you are on purpose.

You do not have to quit your job if you realize you are off course. You can use your current job to fuel your passion. Your passion also does not have to be your job. You can do both. Lose the either-or mentality in life and add the "ands." I can take care of my family *and* pursue my passion. I can make my passion my career. There are no limits, as long as you believe you can do it. You can also bring passion and purpose into your current job. The possibilities are endless. If you do decide to quit your job, believe you will be okay. Have faith that opportunity will come when you open yourself up to it. Do not wait until you are so depressed in your current job that you shut your soul down because you feel stuck due to responsibilities. Do not become immobilized. You can change any situation in your life when you recognize the limiting beliefs and excuses keeping you stuck. Become aware of the connection of your emotions to your higher self and learn new tools to make the changes your soul is craving.

This part of the book will help you get more in touch with your passion and purpose, as well as bring you into alignment with source. Fueling the spirit is a fundamental step in healing. Spend some time exploring where your passions lie and incorporate your passions into your life. The meditations in this book will help you dissociate from the body, tap into your body's healing energy, lower the stress response, heal emotional trauma, sleep better, and create peace.

How to Meditate

Many people feel that because they cannot turn off their thoughts when meditating, they are failing. The ego and our thoughts dominate our minds. The ego wants to be right, so it will show you that thoughts will keep coming and try to convince you that you cannot meditate. When we feel we are not good at something, we give up. It is normal for you to not be able to turn off your thoughts. The thoughts will always be there, some days more than others. Meditation is the act of becoming the observer and getting in touch with your higher self. The ego will resist this, but there is no failing in meditation. Just setting the intention and taking the time to do it is a success. Blaise Pascal says, "All of humanity's troubles stem from man's inability to sit quietly in a room alone." The ego will create excuses like, "I do not have enough time," "I am not good at it," "I cannot turn off my thoughts," and, "It is too hard." Recognize these types of excuses as the ego trying to keep itself alive and in control. We gave up excuses when we started taking responsibility for our lives. Move forward anyway.

The ego wants to be separate. It wants to be identified by its roles. Paramahansa Yogananda said, "Man has falsely identified himself with the ego. When he transfers his sense of identity to his true being, the immortal Soul, he discovers that all pain is unreal. He no longer can even imagine a state of suffering." This is a goal of meditation.

Meditation is not this: You are sitting in your quiet place. You finally feel you have reached a state of calmness and inner peace. It feels wonderful. Then your spouse opens the door and asks you where you put his shirt. You respond in anger, "Would you be quiet? You just ruined my Zen." You get so angry at the interruption that you cannot calm back down.

The practice of meditation is meant to bring peace into everyday moments. Through it, you can learn to respond to interruptions with peace. At the beginning of every meditation, there will be a reminder about interruptions. It will remind you to become the observer of the interruption and the feelings that arise from it. It will also remind you that the goal of meditation is peace, and to bring this peace to your response to the interruption.

If you feel you do not have time to meditate, the first step is replacing the words, "I cannot commit to a meditation practice," or, "I do not have time," with, "I can commit to meditation," and, "I will make time." There was a time when I did not believe I could be a mom and run a business. Jack Canfield taught me to lose the either-or idea and to use the word "and," instead. Practice saying it: "I can run a business and be a mom and write a book and have hobbies and be a wife and practice self-care." When you believe you can, the how will show up. Start changing your limiting language to empowering language and watch your world change. "I can easily make time for a meditation practice," is a great affirmation. Review the "Empowering Language" and "Self-Care and Self-Management" sections in "Part Two: Mind."

The Benefits of Meditation

- ☐ Helps you learn to become the observer.
- ☐ Activates the Laws of Attraction.
- ☐ Puts your body into a state of relaxation needed to heal.
- ☐ Shifts your vibration by connecting you to your higher self and source.
- ☐ Quiets the mind.
- ☐ Helps decrease pain by dissociating with it.
- ☐ Gets you in touch with your passion and purpose.
- ☐ Helps to recharge and energize the body.
- ☐ Increases concentration and focusing skills.
- ☐ Aids in healing post-traumatic stress disorder.
- ☐ Helps you face your fears and gain confidence through mental rehearsal.
- ☐ Promotes spiritual growth.
- ☐ Increases feelings of joy, love, and peace.
- ☐ Promotes better sleep and helps relieve insomnia.
- ☐ Creates integration in the brain.

Types of Meditation

There are hundreds of types of meditations. We can break them down into three generalized forms. The first is focused-attention meditation. In focused-attention meditation, attention and focus are put onto the breath, parts of the body, sounds, or a visualization of an object. Most types of meditation, like Zen, Samatha, Chakra, Qigong, and Mantra Meditation, all fall under this form. The second form of meditation is awareness or observer meditation. This is where the external environment, body, and thoughts are all observed without judgment. They are allowed to come and go. Vipassana and Mindfulness Meditation are the most common forms of awareness meditation. The third form of meditation is that of effortless presence, where attention is put onto oneself. It is a more advanced meditation that often requires prior mental training to achieve.

The meditations I use are a combination of focused attention and awareness meditation. They come from the following traditional forms.

Zazen or Zen is a Buddhist meditation. It is done in a seated position with the back straight. The goal is to see the body, breath, and mind as one. Breathing is done in a relaxed, normal rhythm with focus on the breath. One can steady awareness on the breath by counting. Each combination of inhalation and exhalation is a count of one. It is practiced by counting to ten, then counting back down to one, and repeating the sequence. Whenever a thought interrupts the meditation, you notice it and begin again at one. Thoughts and emotions are not suppressed. The attention is just shifted back to the breath.

Samatha is a Buddhist meditation that focuses on the breath to calm the mind. It is training your attention through concentration. When the mind wanders, you direct it back to the breath.

Vipassana is a Buddhist meditation. It means "insight" or "clear seeing." For this meditation, the back should not be supported. All focus is put on the breath, either through the movement of the belly or the movement of the nostrils. When sensations and thoughts arise in the body and mind, awareness is brought back to the sensation of the breath. There are Vipassana meditation schools where you practice meditation daily and spend ten days or longer in complete silence.

Metta Meditation or Loving Kindness Meditation is a Buddhist meditation that uses focused attention on feelings of love, compassion, kindness, and joy toward oneself, a loved one, a neutral person, a difficult person, and the planet. Practicing this meditation improves one's ability to empathize, increases self-worth, promotes forgiveness, and creates a positive emotional state.

Mindfulness is a Buddhist meditation that focuses on the present moment. Awareness is brought to sensations, thoughts, emotions, breath, and the external environment. One can also practice mindfulness in daily activities by becoming deeply present and only focusing on the moment. For example, when eating, the focus is put onto the smell, the taste, the muscles used to eat, and the sounds around you. It gets you out of the automatic responses that occur when lost in thought and habit.

Mantra Meditation is a Hindu meditation that uses a symbol or word that is repeated as a means to focus your mind. Affirmations are not mantras. Often 108 or 1008 repetitions are used in a standard practice. Many people find it is easier to focus on a word than on the breath. It is great for when the mind is in overdrive and cannot calm with focus on the breath.

Taoist Meditation is a Chinese meditation that includes several types of meditation that generally focus on insight, concentration, and visualizations. A common practice is to visualize the cosmos in relation to oneself. Breathing meditations like Qigong are Taoist meditations that focus on patterns of inhalation and exhalation. Inner Vision is a Taoist meditation that involves visualizations of the inner body, the organs, and energy.

Creating a Meditation Space

For some people, creating a space to meditate can really help with developing a new habit and bringing motivation to meditate. Creating a space can also aid in bringing a healing, inspiring, and peaceful energy into the house. A meditation space can be set up anywhere in the house. Some people will dedicate a room for meditation. Some will make a space in an area of a room. There is no right or wrong. Pictures of spiritual leaders, inspiring quotes, crystals, essential oils, and candles are all great things to add to this space, if you feel creating this area would benefit you. Personally, I do not have a meditation room or space. This is okay too. I meditate anywhere in my house, usually in my bed as Kaiden sleeps, as that is where I have the most time to meditate. Since we co-sleep, it is the perfect place. If you do feel like creating a space, it is best to set the intention to make the space but still start on your meditations as you are creating and collecting objects for the space. Allow it to change and evolve as you add to it and as you begin your practice.

You can also meditate outdoors. Meditating outside is my favorite. One of my greatest pleasures in life is to go into the woods with my dogs, find a sunny spot, and sit and listen. I listen to the sounds of the birds, the trains, and the water if I am by the river. I feel the dogs' energy as they move around me. I listen to the wind and feel it caress my skin. If it is winter, I feel the coldness on my face and against my snowsuit as I sit or lie in the snow. Do what feels best for you.

Creating a New Habit

It takes around thirty days to create a new habit. When you begin to meditate, aim to do it for thirty days in a row. This will instill the new habit in your mind. If you end up skipping a day after the thirty days in a row is complete, your mind should want to go back to it because it is a habit. If you skip a day in the first thirty days, then start counting again at one. Make it a fun game. Do not get upset if you miss a day. The more you start over, the more it will become a habit, as well.

Following are a list of meditations for you to try. The Waking and Bedtime Meditations are meant to be done daily, upon rising and before bed. Then there are ten core meditations to be done at a set time of day. The time you choose is what works best in your schedule. The mini meditations that follow the daytime core meditation are meant to be used anytime throughout the day when you need to rebalance and raise your vibration. You can use them anytime you feel any lower-frequency vibration. They are one to two minutes long and can be done anywhere. You can do a new core meditation each day or spend a few days to a week or longer on each core meditation before moving on. Once you have done them all, you may find that certain meditations resonate more with you, so do those more frequently. If you are looking for structure, then spend one week on each meditation. After that, you should have them ingrained in your mind and be able to choose a meditation depending on what you need that day.

Waking and Bedtime Meditations Introduction

Upon rising and just before going to sleep are key times to attract your desires in your life. The time before bed will set into motion what you attract from source through the night while you are sleeping. It is the time to refocus from lower-frequency emotions to higher-frequency ones. We are going to do this by going over the entire day and seeing all events that did not go your way or could still be troubling you, go your way. You will use visualizations of seeing them as resolved. Another tool you will use is focusing on your achievements throughout the day. Find ways to be proud of yourself. This increases self-worth and self-love. You will also use breath work and visualizations to relax the body and prepare for sleep.

Many people suffer from insomnia. Sleep mindset is essential to addressing insomnia. Learning to be aware of your thoughts around sleep is one of the key methods to creating a good night's rest. If you are suffering from insomnia, it is also good to work with a practitioner who understands how to balance neurotransmitters, sex hormones, and adrenals, as all of these can contribute to insomnia. Detoxification and pathogens are active through the night, which can cause one to awaken between two and four in the morning. If cortisol spikes at this time, or if the mind starts going into overdrive due to runaway thoughts, going back to sleep can be quite difficult. Our thoughts around sleep, as well as our worries in general, can create anxiety and stimulate a stress response. This is not ideal for sleeping. High cortisol suppresses melatonin, the neurotransmitter responsible for sleep. If you are having trouble sleeping, you may have thoughts like, "I need to sleep or I will be tired, depressed, or anxious tomorrow," "If I do not sleep, my day will be ruined," "I should be asleep now," or, "There is something wrong with me. Why am I not asleep?" All of these thoughts will cause feelings of anger, anxiety, and depression. Society does not help, as we see ads for insomnia on TV that promote medication and make not sleeping seem bad. Any symptom you have is a message from your body telling you that it needs help. It could be an imbalance in one of the areas discussed above, or it could be a message indicating you need to do some work on your mindset and self-growth to address the thoughts preventing you from sleeping.

We want to become aware of our thoughts, as those thoughts create beliefs, and our beliefs create our reality. If you believe you need sleep, you first send out the vibration of not getting sleep, so you will attract more of that. You also send out that you will be tired the next day because you believe it. This will make you be tired the next day. Besides having your thoughts attract what you do not want through the Laws of Attraction, you also increase cortisol with those stressful thoughts. Instead, create beliefs like, "My body will sleep when it is ready," "I can use this awake time during the night to focus on mindset training," and, "I will awake refreshed and full of energy regardless of how I sleep."

If you cannot fall asleep, or if you awaken through the night and are unable to fall back to sleep, turn on a meditation or a mindset book. Meditate, rest, and just be in the present moment. If any thoughts come about the next day, just visualize how you want the day to go.

Upon rising, you are still well-connected to source. In the morning meditation, you will tap into this connection and set your vibration for the day. This is done by focusing on gratitude for all that you are thankful for in your life. We also focus on what you appreciate in a loved one and yourself. Gratitude and appreciation are two of the highest vibrations. In the meditation, you will be asked to pick a person to appreciate. I find this very helpful in repairing conflicts. When you focus on what you love about a person, you will get more of those qualities from them. I most often choose my husband. When you live with someone, you tend to have frustrations, annoyances, and often even deeper lower-frequency emotions like anger and resentment. This practice of appreciation has been vital to creating a loving, stable relationship with my husband.

The amazing thing is that it only takes one person to participate. I find that if I start to feel annoyed during the day, my subconscious will bring up one of his good qualities to focus on. It has really deepened my love for him. Eckhart Tolle and Byron Katie are great resources for repairing relationships through self-awareness. If you find you cannot focus on someone you are currently in conflict with, then choose someone who is easier for you to express appreciation for.

In the morning meditation, you will also set your intention for the day. Your intention is not what you are going to do during the day but how you will feel and how you will choose to respond. *I choose to respond with love. I choose to respond with kindness. I choose to be patient. I choose joy. Today I will be kind and patient.* When prompted, you can listen for a soul word to create your intention. A soul word is a message from your higher self. Let your higher self choose what to focus on for the day by waiting for a word to appear when prompted. If you do not see a word, then pick your intention.

Doing this practice daily will bring peace, love, and joy to your being, which puts you in the optimal state of attracting your desires. It is the state of optimal allowance. Lower-frequency vibrations will only block all the good that is coming to you and those lower vibrations do not feel good. We all want to feel love, peace, and joy. This high vibration also allows the body to heal.

The bedtime meditation is best done while lying in your bed. It is okay if you drift off to sleep. The morning meditation is best done while seated in bed with spine straight and legs crossed or over the bed. You can also do it on the floor or in a chair. It is important to do it soon after you wake up. Doing it lying down in bed may cause you to fall back to sleep. This can cause you to feel more fatigued the next time you wake up.

Remember, if ever you are interrupted by someone or something during a meditation, take a deep breath, notice any emotions that arise, and bring the peace of your meditation into your response. You can start again later.

Waking Meditation

Sit up in a comfortable position, cross-legged or with your legs hanging off your bed. Bring your attention to your breath. Take a deep breath in and visualize white light coming from source energy all around you.

Visualize it moving from your lungs and filling your entire abdomen. On the next inhale, move it down into both legs. On the next inhale, see it filling your chest and back. On the next inhale, move it into your arms. On your next inhale, move it into your head. Feel your entire body filled with white light, fueling every cell and giving you energy for the day.

Allow your breathing to return to normal. Bring to mind everything in your life for which you are grateful. It could be your house, your job, your family, your friends, your spouse, activities you love, or your passions. Hold these images in your mind's eye and feel the feeling of love and gratitude. If your mind wanders, come back again. Affirm, "I am happy and grateful for _____."

Now focus on someone in your life. It can be someone you love or someone you admire. What do you appreciate about them? List all of their positive attributes in your mind.

Now focus on yourself. What are your good qualities that you love and appreciate about yourself? Name those qualities in your mind.

Bring your awareness to your body, your head, shoulders, arms, chest, abdominals, pelvis, and both legs. Feel your whole body's life force. Remember a time where you felt immense love and bring that feeling to your entire body. Allow any ideas or inspiration to come to you. Listen and wait for your soul to give you a word or allow a word to come across the darkness of your eyes. This soul word will be your focus for the day.

Now set your intention for the day. This is not what you will do, but how you will be and feel, like, "I am love, joy, and peace." You can also use your soul word. For example, if you saw the word "kindness" your intention would be, "I will respond with kindness."

Bring your awareness back to your breath, slowly move your arms and legs, and open your eyes. Go on about your day, bringing all the energy and intention from your meditation with you. Ideally, have a whole food breakfast and get the body moving by going for a walk, doing yoga, or stretching.

Bedtime Meditation

When you are ready to go to bed for the night, get into bed and lie on your back. You can use a pillow under your knees to keep the strain off your lower back. Close your eyes and bring your awareness to your breath. We will use the breath to relax each part of the body. Breathe light into the top of your head, your face, and your jaw. As you exhale, feel those areas relax and let out all tension. Breathe light into your neck and shoulders and feel them relax on the exhale. Breathe light into your arms and feel them relax on the exhale. Breathe light into your chest and upper back and feel them relax as you exhale. Breathe light into your abdominals and mid back and feel them relax with your exhale. Breathe light into your pelvis and low back and feel them relax with your exhale. Breathe light into your legs and feel them relax with the exhale. Breathe light into your whole body and feel it relax with the exhale.

Allow your breathing to return to its normal rhythm. Now it is time to go over any troubling events that happened throughout the day. Just rest your awareness lightly on the situation, only enough to bring it to mind. Now see the situation as resolved. If it was an argument with someone, see the situation resolved by visualizing the image of resolution. It could be a hug and feeling of contentment that everything is well between you again. If you are troubled about a project that has not been completed, see the project complete, and feel the sense of achievement. If it is a financial situation that is troubling you, see the situation as resolved by visualizing the stocks increasing, a certain amount in your bank account, or a check coming in the mail. Feel the joy that all is as you want it. By focusing on what we want, just a single image with feeling, we attract that to us. Go through any event or thought that has bothered you throughout the day. Spend time holding the image and feeling of what you desire to happen. Live from the outcome you want. If you get carried away by a thought, simply notice it and return to the resolution.

Take a few deep breaths and search your mind for ways you are proud of yourself for things you did throughout the day. This can be any achievement, big or small. Perhaps you chose a whole food item at lunch, went for a walk, completed a task, said something kind to someone, or helped a friend. Rest your awareness on each memory for five to ten seconds, then move on to another. If you find your mind wandering to things you are not proud of, simply bring a quick image to mind of how you would have preferred to respond with love and kindness and then move on without feelings of guilt or shame. Every lower-frequency feeling is just showing you what you would prefer. When you focus on what you would have preferred to happen, the next time it happens, you will do that instead. Take a deep breath and bask in all of your achievements for the day. Affirm, "I am proud of you."

On your next breath, bring your awareness to your whole body's life force. Allow yourself to sink into your bed. Feel the appreciation and gratitude for this safe place to rest and reconnect with source. Affirm, "I am safe." Set the intention for the perfect night. Affirm, "I will have a perfect night and I will wake up well rested and full of energy."

Allow yourself to drift off to sleep by bringing your focus back to your breath or any of the visualizations in this meditation.

Core Daily Meditations

Inner Joy Meditation Introduction

The purpose of this meditation is to quiet your mind and to find your inner joy. People often seek joy, love, and happiness from the external environment. Once we realize that our joy comes from within, no person, place, thing, or event can take away that joy. We can summon this joy at any time, in any circumstance. It allows us to be happy and peaceful, no matter what is going on around us. This is one of my favorite meditations. With practice, you will be able to feel the joy and spread it throughout your body without bringing up any memory. It is a great energy booster. It connects you to source energy and sets the highest vibration. When choosing a memory of an event you love, do not choose one that also comes with pain. For example, if you are remembering the love of a parent that has passed away, and the memory may first bring love but then triggers unresolved grief, choose another one that brings only love until you have healed. You can choose different memories each time you do the meditation. The mini meditation is great to use throughout the day if you find yourself in a lower-vibration state or facing a stressful event. The more you practice this meditation, the more it will sink in that the love comes from inside you. The more you feel it, the more love you will have for yourself. As Buddha is thought to have said, "You, yourself, as much as anybody in the universe, deserve your love and affection."

We are going to start by finding a comfortable position. You do not need to be in the classic meditation position. My favorite position is relaxed in a chair with back upright. It's best not to lie down, as you may fall asleep. It is possible to even fall asleep when you are sitting up, and that is perfectly okay. It just means you needed a little nap. Next time, try to do this meditation when you are more alert.

Remember, if you are interrupted by someone or something during a meditation, take a deep breath, notice any emotions that arise, and bring the peace of your meditation into your response. You can start again later.

Inner Joy Meditation

Close your eyes and take a few deep breaths. Move your awareness to your breath. Inhale for a count of four, pause for a count of two, exhale for a count of four, and then pause for a count of two before repeating the process.

As you complete your first inhalation, pause before releasing the breath. I want you to observe the stillness between the inhale and the exhale. Just listen and be present. On your next exhalation, again, pause for the count of two seconds, and become present. Allow any sound or disturbance you hear to pass through you. If a thought comes during this time, just listen and then let it pass.

Allow your body to get into the rhythm of inhale for four, pause for two, exhale for four, pause for two, and repeat. Inhale, one, two, three, four. Pause for one, two. Exhale, one, two, three, four. Pause for one, two. You will get to the point where counting is no longer needed. It will be as though you have always breathed this way. Feel your body relax with each breath.

Begin to allow your breathing to follow its natural rhythm. Bring to mind a time when you felt pure joy, love, and happiness. It could be a time when you hugged your children, your partner, your parents, your grandparents, or your siblings. It could be at a family gathering, an event like the birth of a child, getting married, or a trip you took. It could be when you hug your pet. The important part is that this memory should create a feeling of intense love and joy. You may feel butterflies and tingling inside you. Realize now that this feeling did not come from the other person or event; it manifested inside of you. The event may have triggered it, but the feeling comes from within. It is your connection to source, to God, to universal consciousness.

Continue to recall this memory. Scan your body to find the location of the feeling. It could be in your solar plexus, your heart, your pelvis, or your throat. When you have found the location, observe its size, texture, and color. Is it round or square? Soft or hard? Hot or cold? What color is it? Picture it in your mind's eye. Hold the feelings of joy and love that the memory brings. This is your consciousness. This is universal energy. It is pure radiant joy, love, and peace.

Take this feeling and spread it throughout your entire abdominal and chest area. See the light and energy of love and joy filling all of your organs with light. Your liver, your stomach, your intestines, up into your lungs and your heart, into your back, the muscles in your abdominals, your bladder, filling in your entire pelvis with a feeling of love and joy. Observe how these areas now feel.

Bringing again the memory to mind, pull the feeling of love and joy down through your right hip, your glute, down into your thigh, your quads, and your hamstrings. Pull the feeling into your knee, down through your calf, and to your ankle. Fill your entire foot all the way to the tips of each toe. Fill it all with radiant, loving light. It may feel as though your leg is buzzing or tingling as the area is filled. Take a second to notice the difference between the left and the right leg.

Bringing again the memory to mind, pull the feeling of love and joy down through your left buttocks, filling your hip, your glutes, down into your thigh, your quads, and your hamstring. Pull the feeling into your knee, down through your calf and to your ankle. Fill your entire foot all the way to the tips of each toe. Fill it all with radiant, loving light.

Come back again to the center of the love and joy and recall again the memory. Next, begin to pull the light and love into your chest and back. Pull it into your right shoulder, down into your upper arm, into your elbow. Pull it down your forearm, into your hand and into each finger, all the way into your nails and shining through the fingertips. Again, notice the difference between your right arm and your left arm.

Come back again to the center of the joy and love, recall again the memory, and we will do the same thing with the left arm. Pull the energy into your left shoulder, down your left upper arm, into your elbow, down your forearm, into the left hand and all the way to the fingers.

Return again to the center of the joy and love, where that memory and that feeling are originating. Next, pull it up through your neck and fill your entire head. Feel it as it flows through your lips, your nose, and your eyes, into your scalp and your hair. Really observe how your entire body feels as it pulsates with love and joy. Now, take that energy, that light, the feeling of joy, and spread it out around you, completely filling your aura. Notice how big your energy field around your body is. It may be anywhere from a few inches to a few feet. See the shape around you, from the top of your head to the tips of your toes.

Come back again to the center of that emotion, build it up as much as you can, and now expand your aura. Push out the bubble of energy as far as you can, ten to fifteen feet on all sides around your body. Watch as your aura, that bubble of energy, passes through the walls, through the floor. Expand your consciousness outside your body to see all the space that your aura is now filling. This energy provides a protective shield around you, allowing in only high-vibration messages and energy. It repels all lower vibrations. See yourself as a beacon of light.

Come back to your body and focus once again on that memory that fills you with pure joy, love, and happiness. Feel your body pulsating with this energy. Now, very slightly open your eyes. Observe the room around you, while you continue to feel the love and the joy. Continue to feel your body pulsating with this energy, your consciousness. Close your eyes again and realize that this feeling is always there. This is your true self, and this feeling can be summoned at any time.

Bring your attention again to your breath. Inhale for four, pause and listen for two, exhale for four, and pause and listen for two. Feel the coolness of the air in your nostrils as you inhale and exhale. While keeping your eyes closed, slowly move your fingers and your toes. Stretch your limbs. When you are ready, open your eyes. Bring this energy with you throughout your day. Use the mini meditation to help you refocus on it at any time.

Inner Joy Mini Meditation

Close your eyes and take a deep breath. As you inhale, see the breath move to every cell in your body. As you exhale, release all tension and stress. Breathe in, filling your body with energy, and breathe out stress. Breathe in higher vibration and breathe out lower frequencies. Recall a memory where you felt intense love. Feel the area in your body where that love is centered and pull the love down through your core all the way to the tips of your toes. On the next inhale, bring the loving energy from the center to the tips of all your fingers. On the next inhale, pull the loving energy up, filling your entire head. Feel your entire body filled with love. Expand it from the central point out to fill your aura. This love re-centers you to the highest vibration and forms a protective energy around you, repelling all lower vibrations. Affirm in your mind or out loud, if you can, "I am love; I am peace; I am joy." Open your eyes and bring this feeling into your day.

Become the Observer Meditation Introduction

The purpose of this meditation is to become the observer of your external environment, your body, and your thoughts. It is a four-part meditation that takes you through each of those. If you practice becoming the observer in meditation, this will allow you to do it more readily throughout the day when you encounter stressful events. Most of us are just reacting to life. By recognizing we are not our bodies, not our thoughts, and not our emotions, that we are in fact the observer, we can take a step back and respond to events and people in our lives through our connections to our higher selves. This brings peace to our relationships and allows us to create the lives we want. This meditation is also great to help you disassociate from pain and other uncomfortable symptoms in the body. It will also help you learn to hold your seated meditation posture longer.

Naming, judging, and labeling is the ego speaking. The ego needs separation. By becoming the observer, we un-label and un-name. We connect with our higher selves, with universal consciousness, with God. According to Stephen Mitchell's translation, the *Tao* states, "The Tao that can be told is not the eternal Tao. The name that can be named is not the eternal name, the unnamable is the eternally real. Naming is the origin of all particular things. Free from desire, you realize the mystery. Caught in desire, you see only the manifestations. Yet mystery and manifestations arise from the same source." Here again we see the dichotomy of allowing and creating. We will be focusing on un-naming, un-labeling, and just becoming the observer, in perfect allowance like the Tao. Soren Kierkegaard said, "Once you label me, you negate me. I am not what I do, I am not what I have, I am not my roles, I am not my body. When those fall away, I am source."

One way to bring this meditation with you throughout your day and become the observer is when you find yourself faced with an annoyance, take a step back, and just listen. Listen to your thoughts around the annoyance, observe any feelings or emotions it brings up in the body, and practice allowing the annoyance to flow through you. Some examples of things I have worked on are the seat belt alarm dinging when I am driving in a parking lot or down a quiet side road, my husband chewing soft food that does not require teeth noises, my husband picking his nails, and dogs barking. Be aware of thoughts like, "That is annoying, I cannot focus, he should not be doing that," or, "He knows I do not like that and does not care." When those thoughts arise, be aware of them, then let them pass, as well. Feel any emotions that come up, such as anger, resentment, and frustration. Allow them to pass. Ones that I am still working on are smells like cigarette smoke and overwhelming perfume. I find the noises to be much easier, as the smells caused me to have migraines for many years. Though they do not any longer, the feelings and thoughts are quite prominent.

Another way to work on becoming the observer is with annoyances in the body. When you feel an itch, do not scratch it right away. Just observe it. Feel the sensation and try allowing it to pass on its own. If you feel like you have to cough, hold it for a second, and observe the feeling. If you are sitting in a position and feel your body tingling and falling asleep, observe it for a minute or so. For any pain in your body, do the same. Observe it. Observe thoughts like, "What if there is something wrong with me? Maybe I have Lupus or another disease? What if I have a brain tumor? What if I am dying?" Those are all examples of thoughts I have had. Observe those thoughts and how they make you feel. Any fear that comes up is a signal that work needs to be done on the belief underneath the fear. Fear of illness, fear of dying, fear of not being able to work. These fears are an opportunity for you to practice stage-three enlightenment. Get out ahead of the event. It does not mean ignoring the pain. You can still get tested, but the more work you do on meditation, mindfulness, and self-growth, instead of being paralyzed by fear, you will face it peacefully knowing you are able to handle anything that comes your way.

This meditation is intended to be done in a seated position, ideally on the floor or on the ground, as it is meant to be slightly uncomfortable. The uncomfortable feelings and sensations in your body will give you something to observe without emotion. If you feel pain, move to a chair, and make sure to get assessed by a practitioner like a doctor, chiropractor, or physiotherapist to make sure there is not dysfunction that makes a seated meditation position contraindicated.

This is a great meditation to practice outside in nature. You can either sit on the grass or on a towel. I have even done it in the snow in a snowsuit. As you become more advanced in becoming the observer, you may find something crawls on your skin like an ant or a spider, and you are able to observe it without fear or reacting. If you are not comfortable with that, then a chair outside also works.

This meditation does not need to be done in a quiet environment. Noise is welcome, as it allows you to become the observer to that, as well.

Eckhart Tolle tells a story about a student seeking enlightenment. The student asked the master, "How does one find enlightenment?" The master said, "Can you hear that waterfall in the distance?" The student listened and said, "Yes Master, I can hear the waterfall." The master said, "Seek enlightenment there." After a moment, the student asked, "Master, what if I did not hear the waterfall?" The master said, "Seek enlightenment there." The key is to listen. When we listen, the mind becomes quiet.

Remember, if you are interrupted by someone or something during a meditation, take a deep breath, notice any emotions that arise, and bring the peace of your meditation into your response. You can start again later.

Become the Observer Meditation

Get into a seated position on the floor or on a chair. Keep your eyes open and allow your gaze to lightly touch objects in the room without naming them. In the beginning, you will find that the name may arise on its own. That is okay. Continue to move your gaze around, allowing the name to leave. If you have been practicing this meditation for some time, you will be able to rest your gaze on each object longer without a name coming. If you are just starting, it will be easier to keep the gaze moving. Do this for a minute or so.

Now close your eyes and listen to the sounds all around you. If names or thoughts come, allow them to pass, and listen again. If there are other beings, animals, or people in the surrounding area, be it close or far, feel for their energy. Observe without emotion or reaction. Just listen. If you get carried away by a thought, that is okay. When you notice that you have been carried away, return again to listening without reacting to the wandering. Do this for a few minutes.

Now bring your awareness to your body. Feel the life force running through it. It may feel like tingling, buzzing, or heat. Notice it without emotion. Allow any thought to come and fade away as you move your awareness through your body. If it is easier for you, you can start at your feet and work your way up to your head without naming parts. Just move your awareness through your body as you did with your eyes open, resting your gaze lightly on objects at the start of the meditation.

By now you may be feeling some uncomfortable sensations. Just notice them and move on. If you complete the scanning of your entire body, just sit in the awareness of your entire body. Allow any emotion or thought of fear or concern wash away. If you do get carried away by a thought, when you notice that you have been carried away, return again to listening without reacting to the wandering. If you have any pain or other symptoms in your body, just notice them without emotion. Do this for three to five minutes.

Now bring your awareness to the darkness behind your eyes. You may see lights of different colors. Focus here, and ask yourself, "I wonder what my next thought will be?" Now listen and wait for the thought to come. As it comes, observe it, then allow it to pass. Wait and listen for the next thought to come. You may hear someone's voice or have a memory come to mind from your childhood. Your thought may be of something you have to do. Allow it to come and pass, then ask again, "I wonder what my next thought will be?" Again, listen. With practice, you will be able to just sit and listen, and the stream of thought will flow.

Scientifically, we have not been able to determine where thought originates. We cannot see a thought in the brain. Its random nature is much like the randomness of quantum physics. When we are quiet, we can hear the connection to the universal consciousness. Where else could insight and ideas come from? Bring your attention back to the darkness behind your eyes. Any time you get carried away by a thought, refocus on your eyelids, and ask again, "I wonder what my next thought will be?" Then listen. Do this for three to five minutes.

Now move your awareness away from the darkness behind your eyes and to your body as a whole. While you feel your entire body's life energy, expand your awareness to include listening to your surroundings at the same time. Feel the body and listen. Allow any thought to come, notice it, and let it fade away. Stay here for as long as you desire. When you are ready, slowly move your body, bring your awareness back to your breath, and open your eyes. Bring the sense of peace and connection to source with you throughout your day.

Become the Observer Mini Meditation

Close your eyes and bring your attention to your breath. Feel the coolness of the air entering your nostrils as you inhale, and feel your belly expand on the next inhale. Listen to the sounds around you. Allow them to pass through you. Any thoughts that come, allow them to flow away. Observe and feel the inner energy of your body moving your awareness through it without emotion. Do this for one to two minutes. When you are ready, take a deep breath, open your eyes, and bring this peace with you throughout the day.

Healing the Past Meditation Introduction

The purpose of this meditation is to help you release any lower-vibration energy that may be keeping you stuck or blocking abundance. It is best to do this meditation when you are feeling higher-vibration emotions, like love and joy. Doing this meditation once a week is enough, as we do not want to stay too long in the past. When you are constantly revisiting the past, trying to figure it out, and observing events over and over, you will perpetuate that past in the future. When we think of certain things, we get more of those things. Instead, we use techniques like this meditation to go back and heal the event, or see what we needed to see, and to figure out what we would want in the future. See the resolution. It is great to do this meditation before your daily core meditation, as you will be able to use the core meditation to shift to a higher vibration after going into the past.

There usually comes a time when emotional healing of the past comes to a place where you are able to just let it all go. With this comes the realization deep within your being that every event has been perfect and led you to exactly where you are today, which is where you need to be. If you find you are feeling a lot of pain when you think of a past event, use this meditation to help release it. Remember, the problem is in your mind. Everything you experience, every relationship, every person, and every event happens in your mind through the way you perceive it. Then it happens over and over again in your mind as you remember it. Everything is a mental image. If the problem is happening in your mind, the solution is also in your mind. There are no stressful events in the universe. The universe does not need a Valium or an antidepressant. There are only stressful thoughts. Stressful thoughts are messages to tell where healing and growth are needed. This meditation is best done seated in a chair. We want to be comfortable but do not want to fall asleep.

Remember, if ever you are interrupted by someone or something during a meditation, take a deep breath, notice any emotions that arise, and bring the peace of your meditation into your response. You can start again later.

Healing the Past Meditation

Close your eyes and focus on your breath. Feel the coolness as the air enters your nostrils. Focus on the rise and fall of your abdomen with each inhale and exhale. Do this for a few minutes.

What is an area of your life where you are stuck? What are you feeling? Scan your body from head to toes. Where do you feel tension, pain, or numbness? Focus your attention on that sensation. Is it solid or hollow? Wet or dry? Cold or hot? How big is it? What color is it? Is there a feeling inside that sensation?

Go back to the first time you felt it. If you are unable to bring this to mind, ask your subconscious for a number. When this number comes, go back to that time in your life. You can also just go back to the time of the stressful event that is bothering you.

Where are you? Are you alone or is there someone with you? Is there something happening that you do not want to be happening or is there something you want to happen that is not happening?

Become the age you are now and go back to that younger self and counsel them. Tell them what they need to hear. Your younger self may want to ask you for something. Give your younger self whatever they need. Show them how this event can turn out to be positive or a learning experience. Tell them how it made you stronger. Explain to them that anyone who contributed to the event was doing their best with the tools they had at that time. If the younger self needs to hear something from a person at that time, speak to your younger self through that person. Perhaps the person needs to apologize or explain their own circumstances as to why they acted a certain way. Allow the situation to play through how you feel it would have been best for you. Be the space for your younger self to express any emotions that need to come out. When you are ready, say goodbye to your younger self, and tell them you are always there when they need you.

Now go to your higher self and ask for guidance on this situation. How would your higher self look back on your entire life? How did this event and healing from it help you along your spiritual journey? How did finding love and forgiveness for yourself and those involved change you? Receive the guidance. Thank your higher self and know that he or she is here for you at any time.

Come back to present and focus on your breath. Feel the air as it passes through your nostrils and the rise and fall of your belly as you inhale and exhale. Slowly open your eyes. Take some time to write down how you feel about the meditation. Do your regular core meditation for the day to re-center yourself to a higher vibration. There is no mini meditation for the Healing the Past Meditation.

Healing Light Meditation Introduction

The purpose of this meditation is to use energy to direct healing to the body. It is great for relaxation, and this is often one I will do to fall asleep when the bedtime meditation is not enough. I also do it quite often when I have a virus.

This meditation can be done in any position, though I find lying down to be most effective, as you can clearly visualize the body. Doing it in a chair also works. We want the body to be comfortable so that pain or uncomfortable sensations from posture are not occurring. We want to send love to all our health issues, not hate them and fight against them. Any force we apply to the illness only strengthens it. When Byron Katie was visiting a friend with cancer, her friend said, "I love you, Katie." Katie replied, "You do not love me until you love your cancer." That is such a powerful message.

Remember, if ever you are interrupted by someone or something during a meditation, take a deep breath, notice any emotions that arise, and bring the peace of your meditation into your response. You can start again later.

Healing Light Meditation

Get into a comfortable position, either seated in a chair or lying down. Your legs and arms should not be crossed. Close your eyes and take a deep breath. Feel the sensation of the air passing through your nostrils. Feel the rise and fall of your belly as you inhale and exhale. Continue breathing at your natural rhythm.

We will begin by moving our awareness into the body. Rest your awareness on the parts of the body named below, feeling the life energy, and allowing each area to relax. Bring your awareness to your head, left shoulder, left arm, left hand, left arm, left shoulder, chest, right shoulder, right arm, right hand, right arm, right shoulder, chest, abdominal area, pelvis, right hip, right leg, right foot, right leg, right hip, pelvis, left hip, left leg, left foot, left leg, left side of the body, right side of the body, whole body.

As you feel your whole body, become aware that all around you is space. Even yourself and the objects surrounding you are made up of mostly space, when you look at the quantum level. In this space, we have access to source energy. Through your breath, we will channel that energy from source.

Visualize a ball of white, bright blue, or violet light beginning to form from source at the base of your left foot. Your left side is your feminine side, which we receive energy from. See the ball of light growing to the size of a watermelon. You will begin to move the ball of energy into your left foot. The energy remains connected to source and will form a trail throughout your body.

Visualize the ball moving into your left foot, healing, energizing, and nurturing every cell it touches. Allow it to fill your entire foot. Move the ball up into your left ankle, up your calf, into your knee, up your thigh, and into your left hip. See your entire leg filled with healing energy. Move the ball of energy into the left side of your pelvis, the left side of your abdominal area, your organs on your left side, the left side of your back, the left side of your chest, heart, and lungs. Move the ball of energy into your left shoulder to your elbow, forearm, and hand, pull it back up to your shoulder, and continue up to the left side of your neck, jaw, face, and head.

Take a second to become aware of the entire left side of your body. Notice how it feels different than the right side of your body.

Move the ball of light from the left side of your head into the right side. Move it down your face into the right side of your neck, down to your right shoulder, and into your right arm. Pull the light into your elbow and hand, then into each finger. Pull the ball back up your arm into your right shoulder. Fill the right side of your chest, lungs, abdominal area, and organs. Bring the light into your right pelvis and hip. Bring the light down your right leg, into your right knee and calf, and fill your right foot. Feel your entire body full of healing light.

Reconnect the ball of energy to the original source starting point. Visualize again the ball of light at the base of your left foot. Again, move the ball up through your left foot, your left leg, and the left side of your pelvis. Move the ball up through the left side of your body, bathing the left-side organs. Move the light up into the left side of your chest and down your left arm to your left hand. Bring it back up your arm to the left side of your neck and head. Visualize the light moving from the left side of your head to the right and down into the right side of your neck to your shoulder. Move the light down the right arm into the hand and back up to the right shoulder. Move the light down the right side of your body, bathing all the right-side organs, and down into your right pelvis and hip. See the light move down your right leg into your right foot.

Feel again your entire body bathing in healing light. Reconnect the ball of light with the source at the base of the foot. You will move the light up the left side of your body and down your right side one more time. This time, move the light through your body at your own pace. When you come over an area where there is any pain, discomfort, or concern, hold the light there for extra time, allowing the area to take what it needs. When you pass over these areas of concern, affirm in your mind, "I am whole. I am love. I am healthy." Begin now, moving the light up your left side and down into your right.

Finish moving the ball of light through your body. If you have not finished each point that needs healing, come back again today, and focus on those areas. Bring again your awareness to your entire body filled with healing source energy. Feel a sense of gratitude knowing your connection to source is there for you anytime.

Bring your awareness back to your breath. Feel the cool air move through your nostrils. Be aware of the rise and fall of your belly as you inhale and exhale. Slowly wiggle your toes and your hands, stretch your body, and then open your eyes. Feel the energy from source still present in your body.

Healing Light Mini Meditation

Close your eyes and bring your attention to your breath. Feel the coolness of the air entering your nostrils as you inhale. Feel your belly expand

and contract on your next breath. Visualize a ball of light connected to source at the base of your left foot. Move the ball up through your left foot, your left leg, the left side of your pelvis. Move the ball up through the left side of your body, bathing the left-side organs. Move the light up into the left side of your chest and down your left arm to your left hand. Bring it back up your arm, to the left side of your neck and head. Visualize the light moving from the left side of your head to the right side and down into the right side of your neck to your shoulder. Move the light down the right arm into the hand and back up to the right shoulder. Move the light down the right side of your body, bathing all the right-side organs, down into your right pelvis and hip. See the light move down your right leg into your right foot. Feel your whole body filled with relaxing blue light. Take a deep breath then open your eyes, bringing that healing energy with you through the day.

Loving Kindness Meditation Introduction

Loving Kindness, or Metta, Meditation is a great meditation to do to raise your vibration. It is especially helpful during times you feel unworthy, angry, unloved, or any other lower-frequency emotion. We can use unconditional love to shift those lower frequencies to higher ones. It also helps build compassion, forgiveness, and empathy for those toward whom you may feel anger, resentment, or hate. When you first begin this meditation, it is okay to direct your love to only yourself and those you care about deeply. As you progress, include neutral beings, and then slowly include ones who bring up lower-frequency emotions. These feelings indicate where inner work and self-growth are needed, as the lower-vibration feelings can only harm you, not the other person. *A Course in Miracles* reminds us, "You who wants peace can find it in complete forgiveness." Resentment is to resend hate and anger. Any resentment or anger you are feeling is only harming you. Resentment and anger require blaming. When we are blaming someone, we are giving away our power. No one has the ability to make you feel anything. Only you have that power. Your feelings always come from how you perceive the past event in the present moment. Forgiveness is to give forth love. The act of sending love to those you have lower-frequency vibrations toward will help heal the wounds you have suffered and bring peace to your soul. Your path to enlightenment looks first at your anger and hate. Clear the junk out of you and you will be on purpose.

I find it helpful to do this meditation in a comfortable position, such as seated in a chair or laying in bed. This will help keep attention focused on loving kindness, not on how uncomfortable you are.

Remember, if ever you are interrupted by someone or something during a meditation, take a deep breath, notice any emotions that arise, and bring the peace of your meditation into your response. You can start again later.

Loving Kindness Meditation

Get into a comfortable position and close your eyes. Take a deep breath in, bringing your awareness to your breath. Feel the coolness of your breath in your nostrils. Feel the rise and fall of your belly. With each inhale, visualize brilliant blue or white light coming into your nose and down into your belly. Pull the light all throughout your body. Each inhale is like the tide, filling you with loving energy. As you exhale, the tide rolls out, bringing with it all stress. Do this for a few minutes.

As you feel your body relax, bring to mind a time in your life where you felt unconditional love. This can be from a parent, a teacher, a friend, a child, or an animal. If you have trouble bringing to mind a memory, imagine someone feeling this way about you. If you find your mind wanders at any time, simply notice the thought, allow it to flow away, and return again to your field of love.

Hold the memory in your mind and allow the feelings to come. Fill your whole body with love. Repeat the affirmation, "I am safe. I am loved. I am healthy. I am whole." Know in your being that you deserve this love. It is the love of source that God has for every being in the universe. Allow your heart to be bathed in this warm, radiant field. You are worthy, and you are enough. You are perfect as you are. Bask in this feeling as best as you can. Affirm again, "I am safe. I am loved. I am healthy. I am whole."

When this loving energy feels strong around you, if you feel comfortable, bring to mind a being you love. Bring them into your field of loving energy. Bring them into your heart. Surround them in a loving embrace. Bless them with your affirmation: "May you be safe. May you be loved. May you be happy. May you be healthy."

Return again to your memory of intense love. When this energy feels strong around you, bring to mind a neutral being. Send them loving energy and see them filled with love. If you feel comfortable, bring them into your field of loving energy. Bring them into your heart. Surround them in a loving embrace. Bless them with your affirmation: "May you be safe. May you be loved. May you be happy. May you be healthy."

Return again to your memory of intense love. When this loving energy feels strong around you, bring to mind a being who has been involved in a difficult situation with you in the past. Send them loving energy and see them filled with love. If you feel comfortable, bring them into your field of loving energy. Bring them into your heart. Surround them in a loving embrace. Recognize that all beings are doing the best they can with the tools, knowledge, skills, and level of consciousness they have. All beings are loved by source. All beings are loved by God. Bless them with your affirmation: "May you be safe. May you be loved. May you be happy. May you be healthy."

Return again to your memory of intense love. When this loving energy feels strong around you, visualize the planet and all of the beings on Earth. Send the entire planet loving energy and see it filled with love. If you feel comfortable, bring the Earth into your field of loving energy. Bring the Earth into your heart. Surround all beings and the planet in a loving embrace. Bless them with your affirmation: "May you be safe. May you be loved. May you be happy. May you be healthy."

Again, refocus your attention back onto the memory where you felt unconditional love to you from another being. Fill every ounce of your being with this love. Recognize this love comes from within you and you can access it anytime. Affirm again, "I am safe. I am loved. I am healthy. I am whole."

Bring your attention back to your breath. Feel the coolness of the air come into your nostrils and your belly expand and contract with each breath. When you are ready, slowly begin to move your body and open your eyes, feeling the love still with you. Bring the love with you throughout your day.

Loving Kindness Mini Meditation

Close your eyes and bring your attention to your breath. Feel the coolness of the air entering your nostrils as you inhale. Feel your belly expand and relax as you breathe in and out. Recall a time where you felt unconditional love from another person to you. Feel that energy expanding and filling your whole body as if you are in a warm embrace. Bring to mind a person who may need this love right now: a friend, a loved one, a neutral person, a stranger, a person you may have ill feeling toward, or Earth. Send them loving energy. If you are comfortable, bring them into your heart and surround them in the warm embrace of love you feel. Bless them with your affirmation: "May you be safe. May you be loved. May you be happy. May you be healthy." Refocus your mind on the memory of love again, filling your body. Affirm, "I am safe. I am loved. I am healthy. I am whole." Take a deep breath, open your eyes, and bring that love with you throughout the day.

Qigong Meditation Introduction

Qigong is an ancient Chinese practice. The word "*Qi*" means "breath," and "*gong*" means "work." Qi is vital force. It corresponds to "*prana*" in Sanskrit and "spirit" in the western world. Qigong uses breath work, postures, meditation, and guided imagery to use Qi to heal the body and promote long life and vitality.

There are two forms of Qigong. The moving meditation involves postures similar to Tai Chi. Once the postures are learned, attention is moved to the flow of energy within the movements. This form is called Wai Dan. The still meditation known as Nei Dan involves seated meditation, imagery, and breath work. Medical Qigong is used to heal oneself and others. Martial Qigong is used to build physical power. Spiritual Qigong is used to work toward enlightenment. Gary Collins from the Jade Sun School of Tai Chi and Qigong said, "The more free you are in your awareness, the more you can consciously feel what you are; the more you consciously feel what you are, the more you can penetrate this physical experience."

This meditation is a basic Qigong meditation I learned many years ago. It starts with being aware of the breath and then moves to guided imagery to bring balance to the organs. If you are interested in learning more about Qigong, there are many online course options and schools all over the world. It is a lifelong practice in itself, and I have only delved lightly into it. This meditation is one I tend to choose when my thoughts are racing. I find it takes a lot to focus on the rise and fall patterns of my hands on my chest and belly. This concentration allows me to break the thought patterns causing me stress and allows me to find peace. From there, I move into the visualization and can maintain the images more easily with less interruption from other thoughts.

Remember, if ever you are interrupted by someone or something during a meditation, take a deep breath, notice any emotions that arise, and bring the peace of your meditation into your response. You can start again later.

Qigong Meditation

Get into a comfortable position and close your eyes. Place your right hand on your chest at the area of your heart and your left hand on your abdomen around your belly button. Take a deep breath, and inhale into your chest. Focus on only raising your right hand. Continue breathing this way for one to two minutes or so, focusing on the rise and fall of your right hand.

On the next inhale, breathe deeply into your belly. Focus on only raising your left hand. Continue breathing this way for a minute or two, focusing on the rise and fall of your left hand.

On the next breath, fill up your chest first, then breathe deep and fill your belly. First your right hand will raise, and then your left hand. As you exhale, let out first your belly and then your chest. On the exhale, your left hand should fall first and then the right. Inhale, raising the right hand and then the left hand. Exhale, lowering the left and then the right. Inhale, filling the chest then belly. Exhale, emptying the belly and then the chest. Continue breathing this way for three to five minutes.

On the next inhale, fill up your belly first and then your chest. On the exhale, empty your chest and then your belly. Inhale raises the left and then the right, exhale lowers the right and then the left. Inhale raises the belly and then chest. Exhale lowers the chest and then belly. Continue breathing this way for three to five minutes.

Allow your breathing to return to normal. On the next inhale, breathe into your heart. With each inhale, feel source energy filling it with vibrant red light. On each exhale, expel all negative energy. Do this for a minute or so.

On the next inhale, breathe into your liver. With each inhale, feel source energy filling it with bright green light. On each exhale, expel all negative energy. Do this for a minute or so.

On the next inhale, breathe into your stomach. With each inhale, feel source energy filling it with bright yellow light. On each exhale, expel all negative energy. Do this for a minute or so.

On the next inhale, breathe into your lungs. With each inhale, feel source energy filling them with bright white light. On each exhale, expel all negative energy. Do this for a minute or so.

On the next inhale, breathe into your kidneys. With each inhale, feel source energy filling them with bright blue light. On each exhale, expel all negative energy. Do this for a minute or so.

See in your mind's eye all of your organs glowing with vibrant light. Your heart red, your liver green, your stomach yellow, your lungs white, and your kidneys blue. With practice, you will be able to hold them all in unison in the mind.

Bring your awareness to your breath. Feel the coolness on your nostrils and the rise and fall of your belly. When you are ready, open your eyes. Bring the relaxation and healing energy with you throughout the day.

Qigong Mini Meditation

This can be done in any position. Close your eyes. Place your right hand on your chest and your left hand on your belly. Take a few deep breaths. On the next breath, fill up your chest first, then breathe deep and fill your belly. First your right hand will raise and then your left hand. As you exhale, let your belly out first and then your chest. On the exhale, your left hand should fall first and then the right. Inhale, raising the right hand and then left hand. Exhale, lowering the left and then the right. Inhale and fill your chest then your belly, exhale empty the belly and then the chest. Continue breathing this way for one to two minutes, feeling your body relax and your mind quiet. You can switch to having the belly rise first and then the chest on the inhale. On the exhale, lower the chest and then your belly. When you are ready, open your eyes and bring the relaxation with you throughout the day.

Create Your Ideal Life Meditation Introduction

In this meditation, we will focus on relaxing the body and mind to connect with your ideal life in three key areas. This activates the Laws of Attraction by focusing on what you want in detail and with feeling. If you are always focusing on what you do not want, this meditation will help you make the shift. This shift in vibration allows your requests to source to flow to you. Focusing on what you do not want is negative goal setting. Even if you do not believe in the Laws of Attraction, shifting focus to what you want will not only help you feel good, but it will also light a fire under you and motivate you to get what you want. It increases your motivation by creating structural tension in your brain.

When you visualize something that is not present, your brain will work to make it happen. It does this by activating the reticular activating system, which is your mind's filter. Resources to help you succeed are always around you. When you focus on what you do not want and have beliefs of lack, your reticular activating system will only filter in things that hold true with those beliefs. Changing your beliefs and your focus will allow your reticular activating system to filter in resources you need to bring your new beliefs to fruition. Successful people dream big. Do not limit yourself. As the saying goes, "It takes the same amount of energy to dream big as it does to dream small." Let go of the fear of failure and trust that the "how" will show up. Just focus on your end goals and live from there as if they have already manifested. It is great to learn how to turn your visualizations into specific goals and affirmations to be used quickly throughout the day. Review the "Create Your Ideal Life" section in "Part Two: Mind."

If you have trouble focusing on what you want, go back to a time in your life when things were going right. This will activate the same vibration. This meditation can be done seated or lying down. You want to be comfortable.

Remember, if ever you are interrupted by someone or something during a meditation, take a deep breath, notice any emotions that arise, and bring the peace of your meditation into your response. You can start again later.

Create Your Ideal Life Meditation

Get into a comfortable position. Bring your awareness to your breath. We will begin by relaxing the body and focusing the mind. With each inhale, you will be contracting a group of muscles then relaxing them on the exhale, allowing the area to sink into the direction of the ground. Start with the muscles of your face and jaw. Contract them on the inhale and relax on the exhale. On the next inhale, contract your neck, and relax on the exhale. On your next inhale, contract your shoulders and pectorals, and relax on the exhale. On your next inhale, contract your arms and hands, and relax them on the exhale. On the next inhale, contract your abdominals and back, and relax on the exhale. On your next inhale, contract your pelvis and hips, and relax them on the exhale. On your next inhale, contract your legs and feet, and relax them on the exhale. Contract the whole body on your next inhale and relax it completely as you exhale.

Take a few deep breaths and bring your awareness to what your ideal financial life and career look like. What is your ideal annual income? How much money do you have in savings? What is your total net worth? Where are you working? What are you doing? With whom are you working? What kind of clients or customers do you have? Is it your own business? Visualize this in detail. How do you feel? Take three to five minutes to visualize this.

Take a few deep breaths and visualize your ideal health and body. How do you feel? What are you doing in your healthy body? Visualize yourself healthy and what you will be doing and feeling. Do not focus on the illness itself. Avoid using words that reference illness. Visualize in detail for three to five minutes.

Take a few deep breaths and visualize what your ideal relationships and your personal life look like. What are your relationships with your spouse and family like? If you are looking for a relationship, visualize that person's ideal qualities. Who are your friends? What do those friendships feel like? Do you see yourself going back to school, getting training, or growing spiritually? Do you meditate or go on spiritual retreats? Do you want to learn to play an instrument or write a book? What are you doing with your family and friends in the free time you have created for yourself? What hobbies are you pursuing? What kinds of vacations do you take? What do you do for fun? Take three to five minutes to visualize this in detail with feeling.

Return your awareness to your breath. Feel the coolness as it enters your nostrils. Feel your belly expand and contract as you breathe in and out. Slowly move your body and open your eyes. Bring the feeling of your ideal life with you throughout the day. Your vision will motivate and inspire you to get the tools to create it.

Create Your Ideal Life Mini Meditation

Do this meditation whenever you find yourself focusing on things you do not want. Close your eyes and pick an area of your life where you have been focusing on lack. It could be finances, career, a relationship, your health or body, or your personal time. Visualize in detail exactly what you want to create. See it as already happening. Who are you with? What do you see? How do you feel? What goal have you reached? What does your life look like in that area? Spend a moment here, and really feel it as if it is already completed. Feel the gratitude. Take a deep breath and open your eyes. Bring that feeling with you throughout the day, motivating and inspiring you to create it.

Affirmations for Health Meditation Introduction

This meditation is one I used to do every day while I was actively experiencing symptoms of Lupus. It focuses on seeing the areas of the body filled with healing light and uses affirmations of, "I am so happy and grateful my body is healthy and whole." Specific visualizations are used for each system of the body, using only empowering language so that we think about what we want, not what we do not want. We do not want to say, "I am pain free," because the mind will still see the word "pain." If you say, "Do not think of a purple horse," you will think of a purple horse. Instead, we will use words like "healthy," "energetic," "limber," and "flexible." These words bring about the feeling of health.

Remember, your state of being is your attraction point. If you feel sick, you will attract more of it. If you feel fat and unlikable, it is impossible to attract the opposite. You will only get more of the same. This meditation helps you shift focus to being healthy, and it also brings your awareness to the vast number of tasks your body is doing every second of the day. Your body wants to be healthy. It is trying its very best to get you there. When you realize this, it helps you move from anger toward it to love and gratitude. Every person I know who has healed themselves of chronic illness looks back at their illness and is thankful for it. On the other side, they see how their illness brought about needed change and growth in their life. Everyone has crap in their life. It is your choice if you want to live in it or use it as fertilizer.

This meditation is easiest when lying down. When prompted to visualize areas, the images do not have to be perfect, just a simple awareness of the area is fine. You can always search for a picture of any area of the body you are unsure of and hold that image in your mind's eye during the visualization.

Remember, if ever you are interrupted by someone or something during a meditation, take a deep breath, notice any emotions that arise, and bring the peace of your meditation into your response. You can start again later.

Affirmations for Health Meditation

Bring your awareness to the breath. We will use the breath to relax each part of the body. On the inhale, breathe blue or white light into the area and on the exhale feel the area relaxing. Feel all tension and stress leaving. Breathe into the top of your head, your face, and your jaw. As you exhale, feel those areas relax, and let out all tension. Breathe into your neck and shoulders and feel them relax on each exhale. Breathe into your arms and feel them relax on the exhale. Breathe into your chest and upper back and feel them relax as you exhale. Breathe into your abdominals and mid back and feel them relax with your exhale. Breathe into your pelvis and low back and feel them relax with your exhale. Breathe into your legs and feel them relax with the exhale. Breathe into your whole body and feel it relax with the exhale.

Allow your breathing to go to its own rhythm. Bring your focus to your brain and visualize it full of a healing blue light. Affirm, "I am so happy and grateful that my mind is healthy and clear." Bring your awareness to your respiratory system, starting from your nose and mouth, then into your throat, larynx, and lungs. Visualize your respiratory system filled with healing blue light. Affirm, "I am so happy and grateful I am breathing clearly." Bring your awareness to your detoxification system: your liver, kidneys, bladder, and skin. See them filled with beautiful healing light. Affirm, "I am so happy and grateful my detoxification is functioning optimally." Visualize your digestive system: your teeth, tongue, mouth, esophagus, stomach, intestines, gall bladder, and anus. Visualize your digestive system filled with beautiful blue light. Affirm, "I am so happy and grateful my digestion is strong, and I easily break down and absorb nutrients. All food nourishes me." Visualize your immune system: your bone marrow, spleen, appendix, lymphatic system, pancreas, and blood. Visualize your immune system filled with brilliant healing light. Affirm, "I am so happy and grateful my immune system is strong." Visualize your muscles and joints, fill them with healing blue light. Affirm, "I am so happy and grateful my muscles are strong, and my joints are limber." Visualize your sensory organs: your skin, your eyes, your ears, your nose, and your tongue. Visualize them filled with brilliant healing light. Affirm, "I am so happy and grateful for my awareness of the world." Visualize your reproductive system filled with brilliant healing light. Affirm, "I am so happy and grateful my sexual energy is vital." Visualize your energy system: your thyroid, mitochondria, pancreas, and every cell in your body. Visualize them filled with brilliant blue light. Affirm, "I am happy and grateful I am full of energy. I am fit. I am strong." Visualize your circulatory system: your heart, lungs, and blood vessels. Visualize your circulatory system filled with healing blue light. Affirm, "I am so happy and grateful my blood flows freely to every cell in my body, nourishing and detoxifying me." Visualize your whole body filled with healing blue light. Affirm, "Thank you, body, for all you do. Thank you for carrying around my consciousness and doing the best job you can to always return to a state of health. I will do my part by focusing on raising my vibration to assist you in healing."

Bring your awareness to your breath. Feel the air come in through your nostrils. Feel your belly expand and contract as you breathe in and out. When you are ready, slowly start to move and open your eyes.

Bring your sense of gratitude for your body and all it does with you through your day.

Affirmation for Health Mini Meditation

Close your eyes and bring your attention to your breath. Feel the coolness of the air entering your nostrils as you inhale. Feel your belly expand and contract as you breathe in and out. Visualize a system of your body that you are concerned with and fill it with blue light. See it healthy and whole. Visualize it filled with healing light. Affirm, "I am so happy and grateful that my _____ is _____." Use your affirmation from the full meditation. Make sure to use empowering language. Feel your whole body filled with healing blue light. "I am so happy and grateful I am healthy and whole. Thank you, body." Take a deep breath, open your eyes, and bring this gratitude with you throughout the day.

Chakra Meditation Introduction

The purpose of this meditation is to unblock, open, and balance your chakras. Chakras are energy centers that belong to the spiritual body and connect us to source energy. "Chakra" is a Sanskrit word that means "wheel" or "cycle." Each chakra corresponds with a different system of the body. When the chakras are open, energy flows and balances the body. Unbalanced chakras contribute to health and emotional issues in the areas of the body to which they correspond. Chakras can be overactive or blocked.

The first chakra, the root chakra, which is located at the base of the spine between the sit bones, corresponds to safety. It is our foundation. It is associated with the color red and the stones bloodstone, garnet, and ruby. Too much activity here is seen as fear and anxiety and often correlates to not having basic needs like food, shelter, safety, and basic emotional needs being met. It deals with survival and is blocked by fear. When blocked, the person may feel disconnected and apathetic. When in balance, you will feel safe and secure in yourself regardless of your current environment and conditions. When balanced, it says, "I am."

The second chakra, the sacral chakra, is located below the belly button and is associated with the color orange and the stones carnelian and citrine. Too much activity here can contribute to addictions and gluttony. Symptoms, including obesity, hormone imbalances, and restlessness, indicate work is needed on the sacral chakra. Blockages can cause depression, impotence, decreased sex drive, and a lack of passion. It deals with pleasure and is blocked by guilt. When in balance, you feel pleasure, balanced sexual energy, and creativity. When balanced, it says, "I feel."

The third chakra, the solar plexus, is located in the area of the stomach, right below the ribcage. It is associated with the color yellow and the stones pyrite, citrine, orange calcite, tiger's eye, and yellow agate. When overactive, you may feel anger, obsessive compulsion, and greed. When underactive, you feel timid, needy, and indecisive. It deals with willpower and is blocked by shame. When in balance, you feel self-confident and powerful, and you have a good sense of self. When balanced, it says, "I do."

The fourth chakra, the heart chakra, is located in the center of your chest at the area of your heart. It is associated with the color green and the stones emerald, rose quartz, and green aventurine. When overactive, it leads to clinginess, putting other people's needs ahead of your own, and a lack of boundaries. When blocked, feelings of heartbreak and the inability to get close to others can be seen. It deals with love and is blocked by grief. When balanced, you feel unconditional love for yourself and others. When balanced, it says, "I love."

The fifth chakra, the throat chakra, is located in the middle of the throat and is associated with the color blue and the stones aquamarine, lapis, and turquoise. When overactive, one may speak loudly and feel they need to be heard. They interrupt others and are said to like the sound of their own voice. When blocked, a person will feel they do not have a voice and suppress their feelings. It is often seen as digestive issues. It deals with truth and is blocked by lies. When balanced, you are able to speak clearly and say your truth with kindness and love. When you speak with a balanced throat chakra, you will enlighten and inspire those around you. When balanced, it says, "I speak."

The sixth chakra, the third eye, is located at the point between the eyebrows. It is associated with the color indigo and the stones amethyst, lapis, and quartz. It is rare for this chakra to be overactive. When it is, it is seen as someone who spends much time in divination and has paranormal experiences. When blocked, you will feel disconnected spiritually and lack intuition. When active, you feel connected to the spiritual world and receive intuition from it without being overwhelmed. An active third eye is a goal of spiritual development. It deals with insight and is blocked by illusion. When balanced, it says, "I see."

The crown chakra is the seventh chakra and is located at the top of the head. It is associated with the color violet and the stones quartz, amethyst, and moonstone. It is said that it is not possible to have an overactive crown chakra. Almost all humans have an underactive one. It is the goal of spiritual growth to activate it, and great spiritual teachers like Jesus, Buddha, Krishna, and others have done so. In our meditations, we still visualize it as being active and balanced. The journey of attempting to achieve this balance brings joy, love, and peace to our lives. It deals with cosmic energy and is blocked by ego attachment. When balanced, it says "I know."

Through meditation, you can balance and unblock the chakras. According to Deepak Chopra, "Each of the seven chakras are governed by spiritual laws, principles of consciousness that we can use to cultivate greater harmony, happiness, and wellbeing in our lives and in the world." I have been doing this meditation since I was a teenager. It is energizing and empowering.

For this meditation, a seated position is preferred, as we desire our root chakra to be in contact with the ground. If you are unable to remain comfortably seated on the floor with legs crossed and a straight back, you can sit on a chair or sit against a couch. If you can do this meditation outside with contact to the earth, that is even more powerful.

Remember, if ever you are interrupted by someone or something during a meditation, take a deep breath, notice any emotions that arise and bring the peace of your meditation into your response. You can start again later.

Chakra Meditation

Get into a comfortable, seated position, and close your eyes. Bring your awareness to your breath. Take a deep breath in, hold it for a second, then breathe out. The counting does not matter. Just take a comfortable deep breath in, hold, and breathe out. Continue this way for a couple of minutes to develop a rhythm. You want the breathing to become natural, as it is the foundation of this meditation.

On your next inhale, see the breath as beautiful white light. This is our connection to source. With each inhale, we are breathing in life-force energy. Observe the light as it comes in through your nostrils and fills your belly.

Now take this light even further. Pull it down to the base of your spine, in between your sit bones. Here you will find your root chakra, a glowing ball of vibrant red light. With each inhale, this ball of red light expands, taking what it needs from source energy. As it expands, see it moving down into the ground, connecting you to the earth and laying strong roots. On your next inhale, affirm out loud or in your mind, "I am secure. I am grounded. I am safe." Your root chakra is now active and strong.

On your next inhale, see the source energy move down into the area below your belly button. Here you will find your sacral chakra, a glowing ball of vibrant orange light. With each inhale, allow your sacral chakra to expand as it takes what it needs from source energy. As source energy fills your sacral chakra, feel your sense of wellbeing, pleasure, and sexuality expanding with it. On your next inhale, affirm, "I am abundant. I am creative." Your sacral chakra is now active and strong.

On your next inhale, move the light from source down into your solar plexus, the area right below the sternum in between your ribs. Your solar plexus is a glowing ball of yellow light. With each inhale, allow your solar plexus to expand and take what it needs from source energy. Feel your self-confidence, self-worth, and willpower rising as it expands. This is your source of power. With your next inhale, affirm, "I am powerful. I am energized. I am enough." Your solar plexus is now active and strong.

On your next inhale, see the energy from source staying at the center of your chest where your heart is located. Here we find your heart chakra, a glowing ball of vibrant green light. With each inhale, allow your heart chakra to expand and take what it needs from source energy. This is your connection to unconditional love. Feel your love for yourself and all others rise as your heart chakra expands. On your next inhale, affirm, "I am love. I am joy. I am peace." Your heart chakra is now active and strong.

On your next inhale, see the light from source energy move into the center of your throat where your throat chakra is located, a glowing ball of bright blue light. With each inhale, allow your throat chakra to expand and take what it needs from source energy. As it expands, so does your ability to communicate your thoughts and emotions clearly and effectively. On your next inhale, affirm, "I speak my truth. I am confident." Your throat chakra is now active and strong.

On your next inhale, see the light from source rising to the point between your eyebrows. Here we find your third eye chakra, a glowing ball of indigo light. With each inhale, allow your third eye to take what it needs from source energy. As it expands, so does your ability to think clearly and make decisions in tune with your highest self. On your next inhale, affirm, "I am wise. I am focused." Your third eye is now active and strong.

On your next inhale, see the light from source rising to your crown chakra right at the top of your head. It is a glowing ball of violet light. With each inhale, allow your crown chakra to expand and take what it needs from source energy. As it expands, feel your connection to your highest self and spirituality deepen. On your next inhale, affirm, "I am connected to my divine self. I am clear." Your crown chakra is now active and strong.

Bring your awareness to your entire body, seeing each chakra glowing and expanding. As the light from each individual chakra expands, all the colors of the rainbow join to create brilliant white light that surrounds your body and fills your aura. With each inhale, the energy and light expand your aura further out from your body. This protects you from all lower-frequency energy that you may encounter throughout the day. While your aura is expanded, you feel all the energies from each chakra strengthen you.

Feel the security, creativity, power, love, confidence, wisdom, and clarity surge though you. Stay here in this feeling for a few moments.

When you are ready, bring your focus back to your breath. Feel the coolness of the air as it fills your nostrils. Feel your belly move up and down with each breath. Slowly wiggle your toes and move your hands. Take as much time as you need to move and stretch your body. When you open your eyes, feel the energy of your chakras. Take this with you throughout your day.

Chakra Mini Meditation

Close your eyes and focus on your breath. As you inhale, see beautiful, vibrant light coming into your nose and filling your belly. Breathe in source energy. Pull this energy down to the base of your spine into your root chakra, a glowing ball of red light. See it expand and take what it needs. On the next inhale, pull source energy down to your sacral chakra below the belly button. Allow the orange ball of light to take what it needs. On the next inhale, pull source energy to your solar plexus at the area of your stomach. Allow this glowing ball of yellow light to take what it needs. On the next inhale, bring the source energy to your heart chakra, allowing the glowing ball of green energy to take what it needs. On the next inhale, bring the source energy to your throat chakra, allowing the glowing ball of blue light to take what it needs. On the next inhale, bring the source energy up to fill your third eye between your eyebrows. Allow this ball of indigo light to take what it needs. On the next inhale, bring the source energy up to your glowing violet crown chakra. Allow it to take what it needs. See all seven chakras glowing with the colors of the rainbow. They coalesce to form bright, white light that fills your aura. Expand your aura around you, raising your vibration and energy and blocking any lower vibrations. Take a deep breath, and open your eyes, bringing this energy with you into your day.

Releasing Pain Meditation Introduction

This meditation is designed to aid in dissociation from pain by recognizing the thoughts and emotions you have toward pain. "Pain happens, suffering is optional," has been quoted by all spiritual leaders. Byron Katie speaks a lot about the pain she had in her life after her transformation, including a heart attack, a car accident, a tumor on her face, crippling neuralgia, and a painful eye disease that nearly took her vision. All through it, she accepted the pain and continued to speak to audiences all over the world from a place of love and joy. Sai Baba, an Indian spiritual master who was regarded by his devotees as a saint, was asked why he did not heal himself from his ailments when he had healed so many others. He said, "My life is my message. People need to give up body attachment and experience divinity within. Pain is a natural phenomenon. Suffering is a choice. I do not suffer; I am not my body."

Pain and other symptoms in the body are not what cause the suffering. The thoughts we have around them are what causes suffering. We may be visualizing a future filled with pain. Thoughts like, "This is never going to end," "My life is ruined," "I cannot live like this," and, "I cannot take much more of this," all project a bleak future of misery. Or our thoughts create a victim mentality, "Why did God do this to me?" "What did I do to deserve this?" "This is not fair." These thoughts are where the suffering comes from.

This meditation is a great first step in becoming aware of your thoughts and emotions toward pain. When you know the thoughts, you can work through them. I recommend doing Byron Katie's *The Work* on these thoughts. The more you practice this meditation, the less reactive you will become to pain and other symptoms in the body.

This meditation is going to feel repetitive. That is purposeful. The conscious mind learns by understanding. The subconscious mind learns through repetition. The more you read, hear, or say the words, the more it will sink in and become true for you. This meditation is best done in a comfortable position, lying down, or seated with support.

Remember, if ever you are interrupted by someone or something during a meditation, take a deep breath, notice any emotions that arise, and bring the peace of your meditation into your response. You can start again later.

Releasing Pain Meditation

Get into a comfortable position and close your eyes. Place your right hand on your chest at the area of your heart and your left hand on your abdomen around your belly button. Take a deep breath and inhale into your chest. Focus on only raising your right hand. Continue breathing this way for one to two minutes or so, focusing on the rise and fall of your right hand. On the next inhale, breathe deeply into your belly. Focus on only raising your left hand. Continue breathing this way for a minute or two, focusing on the rise and fall of your left hand.

Allow your breathing to return to its own rhythm. Bring your awareness into your body and feel how relaxed it is from focusing on your breath. Focus your attention on your left foot and leg. Scan the area for any sources of pain or concern. This could be an injury, pain, or a rash. Rest your attention on this area. Describe it. Is it solid or hollow? Wet or dry? Cold or hot? How big is it? What color is it? Is there a feeling inside that sensation? Quiet your mind and allow any thoughts or feelings you may have around this pain or concern to come to you. Recognize that you are the observer. You are not the pain, and you are not the thoughts. You can choose to put your focus on the sensation, or you can move your awareness to your thoughts. You can also choose your thoughts. Decide now to choose a higher-frequency thought, a healing thought. Affirm, "I am not my body. I am not my thoughts. I am healing. I am whole."

Bring your awareness to your right leg and foot. Scan the area for any sources of pain or concern. Rest your attention on this area. Describe it. Is it solid or hollow? Wet or dry? Cold or hot? How big is it? What color is it? Is there a feeling inside that sensation? Quiet your mind and allow any thoughts or feelings you may have around this pain or concern to come. Recognize again that you are the observer. You are not the pain, and you are not the thoughts. You can choose to put your focus on the sensation, or you can move your awareness to your thoughts. You can also choose your thoughts. Decide now to choose a higher-frequency thought, a healing thought. Affirm, "I am not my body. I am not my thoughts. I am healing. I am whole."

Bring your awareness to your pelvis, low back, and organs in that area. Scan the area for any sources of pain or concern. This could be an injury, pain, or a rash. Rest your attention on this area. Describe it. Is it solid or hollow? Wet or dry? Cold or hot? How big is it? What color is it? Is there a feeling inside that sensation? Quiet your mind and allow any thoughts or feelings you may have around this pain or concern to come. Recognize that you are the observer. You are not the pain, and you are not the thoughts. You can choose to put your focus on the sensation, or you can move your awareness to your thoughts. You can also choose your thoughts. Decide now to choose a higher-frequency thought, a healing thought. Affirm, "I am not my body. I am not my thoughts. I am healing. I am whole."

Bring your awareness to your abdomen and mid back and organs in that area. Scan the area for any sources of pain or concern. Rest your attention on this area. Describe it. Is it solid or hollow? Wet or dry? Cold or hot? How big is it? What color is it? Is there a feeling inside that sensation? Quiet your mind and allow any thoughts or feelings you may have around this pain or concern to come. Recognize that you are the observer. You are not the pain, and you are not the thoughts. You can choose to put your focus on the sensation, or you can move your awareness to your thoughts. You can also choose your thoughts. Decide now to choose a higher-frequency thought, a healing thought. Affirm, "I am not my body. I am not my thoughts. I am healing. I am whole."

Bring your awareness to your chest and upper back and any organs in the area. Scan the area for any sources of pain or concern. Rest your attention on this area. Describe it. Is it solid or hollow? Wet or dry? Cold or hot? How big is it? What color is it? Is there a feeling inside that sensation? Quiet your mind and allow any thoughts or feelings you may have around this pain or concern to come. Recognize that you are the observer. You are not the pain, and you are not the thoughts. You can choose to put your focus on the sensation, or you can move your awareness to your thoughts. You can also choose your thoughts. Decide now to choose a higher-frequency thought, a healing thought. Affirm, "I am not my body. I am not my thoughts. I am healing. I am whole."

Bring your awareness to your left arm and shoulder. Scan the area for any sources of pain or concern. Rest your attention on this area. Describe it. Is it solid or hollow? Wet or dry? Cold or hot? How big is it? What color is it? Is there a feeling inside that sensation? Quiet your mind and allow any thoughts or feelings you may have around this pain or concern to come. Recognize that you are the observer. You are not the pain, and you are not the thoughts. You can choose to put your focus on the sensation, or you can move your awareness to your thoughts. You can also choose your thoughts. Decide now to choose a higher-frequency thought, a healing thought. Affirm, "I am not my body. I am not my thoughts. I am healing. I am whole."

Bring your awareness to your right arm and shoulder. Scan the area for any sources of pain or concern. Rest your attention on this area. Describe it. Is it solid or hollow? Wet or dry? Cold or hot? How big is it? What color is it? Is there a feeling inside that sensation? Quiet your mind and allow any thoughts or feelings you may have around this pain or concern to come. Recognize that you are the observer. You are not the pain, and you are not the thoughts. You can choose to put your focus on the sensation, or you can move your awareness to your thoughts. You can also choose your thoughts. Decide now to choose a higher-frequency thought, a healing thought. Affirm, "I am not my body. I am not my thoughts. I am healing. I am whole."

Bring your awareness to your neck and head. Scan the area for any sources of pain or concern. Rest your attention on this area. Describe it.

Is it solid or hollow? Wet or dry? Cold or hot? How big is it? What color is it? Is there a feeling inside that sensation? Quiet your mind and allow any thoughts or feelings you may have around this pain or concern to come. Recognize that you are the observer. You are not the pain, and you are not the thoughts. You can choose to put your focus on the sensation, or you can move your awareness to your thoughts. You can also choose your thoughts. Decide now to choose a higher-frequency thought, a healing thought. Affirm, "I am not my body. I am not my thoughts. I am healing. I am whole."

Take a deep breath and fill your body with healing blue light. Feel the power you have to move your awareness to anything you like, the power to choose your thoughts. Slowly begin to move your body, open your eyes, and bring this feeling with you throughout your day. When events happen, take a step back, and become the observer. See things from a third party, unbiased perspective. See things as your higher self and respond from there.

Releasing Pain Mini Meditation

Close your eyes and take a few deep breaths. Scan your body for any sources of pain or concern. It could be an injury, pain, or a rash. Rest your attention on this area. Describe it. Is it solid or hollow? Wet or dry? Cold or hot? How big is it? What color is it? Is there a feeling inside that sensation? Quiet your mind and allow any thoughts or feelings you may have around this pain or concern to come. Recognize that you are the observer. You are not the pain, and you are not the thoughts. You can choose to put your focus on the sensation, or you can move your awareness to your thoughts. You can also choose your thoughts. Decide now to choose a higher-frequency thought, a healing thought. Affirm, "I am not my body, I am not my thoughts. I am healing, I am whole."

Take a deep breath and fill your body with healing blue light. Feel the power you have to move your awareness to anything you like, the power to choose your thoughts. Slowly begin to move your body, open your eyes, and bring this feeling with you throughout your day.

Cosmic Sound Meditation Introduction

The purpose of this meditation is to energize and relax your body at the same time. It brings deep stillness to the mind along with immense power. It connects you to source. It can be done in any position, lying down, or sitting. The beginning of the meditation includes visualization of the quantum state and the cosmic universe. Visualizing the scope of the universe and the creation possible from the one divine mind that we are connected to shows that any problem of today's world can easily be solved with the right mindset. God said, "I am that I am." (Exodus 3:14 KJV) What He meant is, "I am that. I am that. I am that." He is everything. That means He is in you. You are one with God. One with source. You have access to the infinite creative force. The sound "AHHH" is the sound of God. You can hear it in all of His names: God, Krishna, Buddha, or Allah. Repeating the sound of God is called Japa Meditation, and is found in Hinduism, Jainism, Sikhism, Buddhism, and Shintoism. The sound "AHHH" requires no effort on our part to produce. If you are not comfortable using "AHHH," you can use the sound "OHM." Since I was young, I have always used the sound "OHM" in my meditations. Recently, I discovered the power of using the sound of God in Wayne Dyer's books and now use it more often than OHM. Wayne Dyer said, "Sounds have the power to generate your ability to attract to yourself that which you desire. Sounds have power."

Remember, if ever you are interrupted by someone or something during a meditation, take a deep breath, notice any emotions that arise, and bring the peace of your meditation into your response. You can start again later.

Cosmic Sound Meditation

Bring your awareness to the breath. We will use the breath to relax each part of the body. Breathe into the top of your head, your face and jaw. As you exhale, feel those areas relax and let out all tension. Breathe into your neck and shoulders and feel them relax as you exhale. Breathe into your arms and feel them relax on the exhale. Breathe into your chest and upper back and feel them relax as you exhale. Breathe into your abdominals and mid back and feel them relax with your exhale. Breathe into your pelvis and low back and feel them relax with your exhale. Breathe into your legs and feel them relax with your exhale. Breathe into your whole body and feel it relax with the exhale.

Bring your awareness to the darkness behind your eyelids. Allow your eyes to become a lighted microscope and zoom in to see each individual cell of your eyelids. Zoom in further and see the cell's nucleus that contains your DNA. Zoom in further to see the individual base molecules that make up your DNA. Zoom in even further and see the individual atoms that make up those molecules. Zoom in even further and see the electrons. Zoom even further still and you would get all the way down to quanta of energy that are the smallest we can see. Immense space is located between each, just like in the cosmos. These quanta come in and out from connection with source. Every cell of your being is connected to source.

Now bring your awareness back to the space behind your eyelids. Visualize yourself rising up above Earth. From here, you can see the vastness of the world. Rise up further and observe Earth orbiting the sun. Rise up further and see all of the planets circling the sun. Rise up further and see the vast space between stars. Rise up even further still and see the vastness between galaxies and the ever-expanding universe. Think of the billions of years that have passed and the billions that will pass. Feel the awe of the immensity of the universe and the power of the source that created it.

Slowly come back to your body, holding the vastness of the universe and the connection to source in each and every one of your cells. You are part of the oneness. You have access to the creative force of the universe. You have the power to change any situation in your life. Let's connect further with that energy.

Bring your awareness to your breath. Take a breath in, hold, and breath out. Breath in, hold, and breath out. With each inhale, slowly increase the length of your inhale; slow your exhale, pausing slightly in between the inhale and the exhale. Do this for a minute or so to increase your breathing power.

Starting on your next breath, on each inhale, see the words, "I am." On the pause between breaths, go into the space, the connection with source, and as you exhale, say the sound "OHM" or "AHH" out loud if you are able, or in your head if you are not able to out loud. Feel your body filling with a calm, powerful energy as you connect to source. Do this for three to five minutes, or longer if you are able. If you find your mind wandering, just notice it, and come back to the mantra.

Allow your breathing to return to normal. Focus on your body and the sensation of power and peace. Slowly open your eyes and bring that sensation with you. You have the power to create your life.

Cosmic Sound Mini Meditation

Bring your awareness to your breath. Take a breath in, hold, and breathe out. Breath in, hold and breathe out. With each breath, slowly increase the length of your inhale; slow your exhale, pausing slightly between the inhale and the exhale.

Starting on your next breath, on each inhale, see the words, "I am." On the pause between breaths, go into the space, the connection with source, and as you exhale, say "OHM" or "AHHH" out loud if you are able, or in your head if you are not able to. Feel your body filling with a calm, powerful energy as you connect to source. Do this for one to two minutes. If you find your mind wandering, just notice it, and come back to the mantra.

Allow your breathing to return to normal. Focus on your body and the sensation of power and peace. Slowly open your eyes and bring that sensation with you. You have the power to create your life. Bring this feeling with you throughout your day.

Continuing Your Meditation Routine

Meditation is a key part of my self-care routine. My hope after reading this book and doing the meditations is that you are able to really feel the benefits of meditation for yourself, and that you are able to become the observer of your thoughts, body, and environment. I hope you are able to use meditation to activate the Laws of Attraction in your life to attract your desires, and that you are able to use meditation to shift your vibration to promote healing and connect to source. I hope you are finding your concentration and memory have started to improve, you are able to use meditation to promote sleep and energize the body, and you are starting to feel a greater sense of joy, peace, and love. I hope you continue to develop all of these skills through meditation and include meditation as a key part of your self-care routine.

After doing the meditations for thirty days, it should be a habit, or very close to a habit. Even if you skip days, your mind should yearn for it and return to it as soon as possible. If you find that there are days when you are unable to complete a longer meditation, the mini meditations are great to keep you centered throughout the day. Of course, it is very easy to get in the morning and evening meditation routine. These will give you a good base of vibration and attraction throughout the day. You can continue to do the meditations for another thirty days or pick and choose your favorite meditations based on what you need that day.

A Gift We Can Give Our Planet

Another reason I hope you continue your meditation routine is because I feel it is vital for our planet. We know that no amount of being angry or sad at the suffering or problems of the world can change what is going on. No matter how sad we are that people are starving in other countries, it will not bring them food. Those vibrations of anger and sadness will only bring more things that cause anger and sadness. Even if you send money, it will not do much good if you send it while in a state of sadness. If you send money for a charitable cause, make sure you send it while you are operating from a higher-vibration state, as not only will you help the charities, but you also will have an effect on the world, itself.

Water forms beautiful crystalline structures. This structure is destroyed by the chemicals and processes used in the sanitization process. We can use quartz crystals and devices like the Somavedic to restructure water back into crystalline form. Experiments have shown that our thoughts can also restructure water over time. Speaking high-frequency words of love and peace to water will cause it to begin to restructure. Speaking low-frequency words that send out anger and hate will not. Also, if the water is already in crystalline form, those lower-frequency words will cause it to lose its structure. That is how powerful a single person's thoughts are. We are made mostly of water. Our planet is made mostly of water. Imagine how our combined thoughts are affecting the energy of our planet.

The best gift we can give our planet is working to live in a vibration of peace and love. If all humans were emitting mostly love and peaceful vibrations, we could restructure the world. If all of humanity took the time to focus on self-growth, spirituality, and mindset work, imagine the world we could create. Perhaps contrast is only necessary to create that world. I see our planet and all the beings on it as a single organism. Humans can either be pathogens, fighting each other and destroying the host along with each other; or we can be one with the planet, working to nurture it and grow. One cannot meet any of the world's issues with anger, resentment, and hate. That only brings more of it. First, we must finish the war going on in our own bodies and minds. End the violence that is there. Be in a state of allowance for what is happening within you and in the world, while believing in your ability to influence your surroundings. Raise your vibration to these higher levels of consciousness, Heal Yourself, Body, Mind, and Spirit, and help change the world.

APPENDIX

Detoxification Pathways

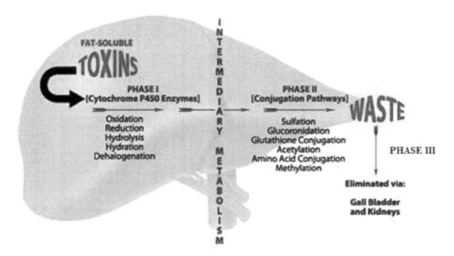

Figure One: Image from http://balancedconcepts.
net/liver_phases_detox_paths.pdf

Phase One Detoxification

Phase one detoxification mostly uses enzymes called cytochrome p450 (CYP) to break down toxins into smaller units using oxidation (adds an oxygen molecule), reduction (removes oxygen), or hydrolysis (adding a water molecule). Some toxins are immediately excreted after going through phase one. The remaining toxins go to phase two detoxification.

Phase one prepares the toxins for phase two. After going through phase one, some of the by-products are more toxic than the original and need to get through phase two immediately. When you have mutations on CYP enzymes, they will function slower, which means it will take you longer to break down different toxins, hormones, medications, etc. Toxins will build up in the body. If you do not have mutations, your phase one enzymes can function too quickly for your phase two to keep up with, especially when there is dysfunction in phase two. Often this presents as multiple food and chemical sensitivities. When this is the case, we want to slow down phase one temporarily and speed up phase two.

To speed up phase one, use indoles from cruciferous vegetables: cabbage, broccoli, and Brussels sprouts. B vitamins, NAC (N-acetyl cysteine), caraway, dill, vitamin C, flavonoids, choline, and inositol also increase the speed of phase one enzymes. Before adding in high amounts of sulfur, rule out sulfur issues like CBS (cystathionine beta-synthase) and MTHFR (Methylenetetrahydrofolate reductase) A1298C mutations, as well as hydrogen sulfide SIBO. See "Genetics Test Analysis" section.

If phase one is moving too quickly, it can be slowed down using grapefruit juice, curcumin, capsaicin, clove, quercetin, and milk thistle. Slowing down phase one is only meant to be done for short periods to allow phase two to catch up.

Phase Two Detoxification

Phase two detoxification is composed of six pathways. Phase two involves converting the toxins from phase one into water-soluble and fat-soluble substances that can then be eliminated safely through urine and bile. The seven phases are:

1. The sulfation pathway
2. The glucuronidation pathway
3. The glutathione conjugation pathway
4. The acetylation pathway
5. The amino acid conjugation pathway

6. The methylation pathway
7. The sulfoxidation pathway

The Sulfation Pathway

Toxins are prepared for elimination by attaching a sulfate molecule to them. When there is inadequate sulfate, toxins and metabolites can accumulate. Sulfate is used to detoxify many substances, including: adrenal and thyroid hormones, salicylates, aspirin, food additives, neurotransmitters, cortisol, many drugs and environmental toxins, and phenols. Symptoms of dysfunction in sulfation include sensitivities to salicylates, phenols, aspirin, and food coloring. Phenols are found in many of the foods we eat, like fruits, veggies, and nuts. They can also be found in products such as toothpaste, hair dyes, medicine, and disinfectants. Salicylates are a type of phenol. High levels of salicylates are found in apples, apricots, berries, oranges, nectarines, grapes, peaches, plums, cucumbers, tea, and tomatoes.

We can become low in sulfate due to intestinal bacteria using up the pathway or a problem with sulfoxidation, which is the ability to convert sulfur in food to sulfate. On the DUTCH Test, we see DHEA (dehydroepiandrosterone) and DHEAS levels. The S is the addition of sulfate to DHEA, to metabolize it. If DHEA levels are much higher than DHEAS, it indicates decreased sulfation.

Increasing sulfation after it has been impaired for a long time can create a detoxification reaction. Adding in sulfur rich foods and supplements is the best way to increase sulfation. Doing this is contraindicated with an active CBS mutation and hydrogen sulfide SIBO. I have also found many people with MTHFR A1298C mutations do not tolerate high sulfur foods and sulfur supplements in high doses. Slow and steady is the key and listen to the body for issues. It is best not to push past detoxification reactions. High sulfur foods include: broccoli, cauliflower, Brussels sprouts, eggs, nuts, seeds, garlic, onion, and asparagus. Sulfur rich supplements include: methionine, taurine, Epsom salts, MSM (methylsulfonylmethane), glutathione, NAC, and glucosamine sulfate. If there are issues with sulfoxidation, it is best to use sulfur sources that are already in the form of sulfate like glucosamine sulfate and Epsom salt baths. Non-steroidal anti-inflammatory drugs (aspirin), and tartrazine (yellow food dye) will deplete sulfate levels. To heal this pathway, reduce intake of salicylates, phenols, and sulfites while working on adding in sulfate. As you rebuild sulfate levels, you can add the foods back in.

The Glucuronidation Pathway

Glucuronidation is the combining of glucuronic acid with toxins using the enzyme UDP glucuronyl transferase (UDPGT). Glucuronic acid is made from glucose. This is a secondary pathway for the most part, as sulfation and glycination are quicker. Glucuronidation will pick up the slack when those two are saturated or damaged.

Glucuronidation helps detoxify substances like pollutants, fatty acids, vitamin A, bile acids, bilirubin, aspirin, benzodiazepines, aspartame, phenols, alcohols, thiols, sulfa drugs, amines, menthol, preservatives, adrenal hormones, androgens, and estrogens. Glucuronidation requires magnesium and B vitamins to function.

Oxidative damage from free radicals damages this pathway. When the main detoxification pathways are damaged, glucuronidation will eventually become overloaded, as well. Glucuronidation does not work well in people with Gilbert's Syndrome. People with Gilbert's have a high level of bilirubin in the blood. Bilirubin is produced by the breakdown of red blood cells, and it then goes to the liver to be processed in this pathway. Normally people with Gilbert's have no symptoms, but some will have fatigue and yellowish skin and eyes. You can increase the UDPGT activity with limonene from citrus peel, dill weed oil, and caraway oil, along with methionine and SAMe (S-adenosyl-L-methionine). Use caution with the latter if you have CBS and COMT (Catechol-O-methyltransferase) mutations.

Glutathione Conjugation Pathway

This is a primary phase two detoxification route that adds glutathione to a substance to detoxify it. Glutathione contains cysteine, glutamic acid, and glycine. Its production requires magnesium, selenium, vitamin B2, and zinc.

Glutathione is used to detoxify heavy metals, herbicides, fungicides, and hydrocarbons. Exposure to these toxins will decrease its levels significantly. When glutathione levels are decreased, toxic burden and oxidant levels increase, as it is a major antioxidant and is needed to regenerate vitamin C and vitamin E.

Nutrients that help increase glutathione levels include vitamin C, alpha-lipoic acid, whey protein, and the amino acids glutamine, methionine, and cysteine.

Smoking burns through glutathione, both in the detoxification of nicotine and in the neutralization of free radicals produced by the toxins in the smoke. Avoid exposure to herbicides, fungicides, insect sprays, and industrial solvents.

Food sources of glutathione are fresh fruits and vegetables, cooked fish, cruciferous veggies, and meat. Supplements to increase glutathione include vitamin C, vitamin E, NAC, and reduced and liposomal glutathione. Coffee enemas have been shown to increase glutathione levels significantly. Glutathione levels are measured on the Organic Acids Test and DUTCH Test. Both high and low metabolite levels indicate a need for support. Before supplementing with vitamin E, check for a GSTP (Glutathione S-transferase) mutation. A mutation here will make it harder to break down alpha tocopherol, the most common vitamin E supplement. If you have a mutation, it is best to get vitamin E from whole food sources like avocado or supplement with tocotrienols.

Acetylation Pathway

In this pathway, detoxification occurs by attaching acetyl-CoA to a toxin using the enzyme N-acetyl Transferase. This pathway requires vitamin B5 (pantothenic acid), vitamin B1 (thiamine), and vitamin C as cofactors. Acetylation detoxifies sulfa drugs, many other antibiotics, histamine, serotonin, and salicylic acid. It also detoxifies many environmental toxins, including tobacco smoke and exhaust fumes.

When there is dysfunction in acetylation, it decreases bile production, which results in the poor absorption of fats and fat-soluble vitamins. Slow acetylators have a buildup of toxins in the system. When this pathway functions too quickly, it is not good either, as fast acetylators add acetyl groups so rapidly that they make mistakes in the process. Both slow and fast acetylators are at increased risk for toxic overload if they are exposed to environmental toxins. If the toxin exposure is reduced, the risk is reduced. Check your genetics for NAT (N-acetyltransferase) 2 mutations. Running your 23andMe through the gene reader Nutrahacker will show you if you have increased, decreased, or normal acetylation.

Consumption of most vegetables and fruits, but especially cruciferous vegetables, increases acetylation, as does glycine, vitamin B5, thiamine, and vitamin C. When acetylation is slow, it is important to support with bile salts at the end of fatty meals.

Amino Acid Conjugation

This pathway attaches an amino acid to a substance to detoxify it. Glycine, taurine, glutamine, arginine, and ornithine will be highlighted.

Glycination is the addition of glycine. It is used primarily to detoxify salicylates and benzoates. Toxin overload will cause glycine deficiency, as will leaky gut and poor protein absorption. People suffering from hepatitis, alcoholic liver disorders, cancer, chronic arthritis, hypothyroidism, toxemia during pregnancy, and excessive chemical exposure are commonly found to have a poorly functioning amino acid conjugation system. Low protein diets will cause deficiency in glycine and other amino acids. Glycine is found in many supplements.

Taurine is a sulfur-containing amino acid that does not cause problems with sulfoxidation but is contraindicated with an active CBS mutation. It is needed to bind with bile in order to excrete toxins.

Glutamine gets huge recognition for gut and mucosal membrane support but is needed for many parts of liver detoxification. Stress in any form will reduce it. The brain makes the neurotransmitters GABA (Gamma aminobutyric acid) and glutamic acid from it. Muscles use it for fuel. It is contraindicated for people with GAD (Glutamic Acid Decarboxylase) mutations.

Arginine is important for detoxifying ammonia in the urea cycle. It is contraindicated for people with herpes virus, as it will activate the virus. Arginine can cause increased blood flow and aid in erections in men.

Ornithine also helps detoxify ammonia to urea. It promotes sleep, so it is best taken at night. It can be converted to arginine. Balance with lysine if you have a history of herpes. Citrulline also helps detoxify ammonia.

The Methylation Pathway

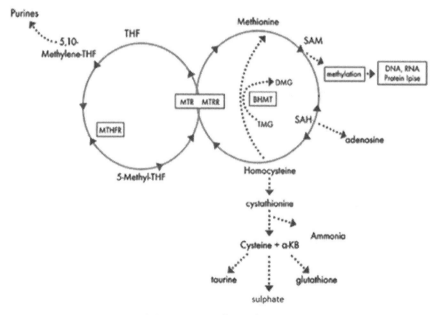

Figure Two: Image from https://www.
greatplainslaboratory.com/dna-methylation

This pathway attaches a methyl group to detoxify many steroid hormones, amines, phenols, thiols, noradrenaline, adrenaline, dopamine, melatonin, L-dopa, histamine, serotonin, pyridine, sulfites, and many other toxins. Adding a methyl group can be used to inactivate viruses, turn on and off genetic mutations, and inactivate cancer cells. It is currently getting a lot of attention with the new understanding of MTHFR gene mutations. It is a complex pathway and requires co-factors vitamin B12, methylfolate (B9), vitamin B6 (P5P), many minerals, and choline. See Figure 2. Methionine is first converted into SAMe, which donates the methyl group, and methylation occurs. The left over SAH (S-adenosylhomocysteine) is converted to homocysteine. Homocysteine can take two routes from there. It can go into transulfuration using the CBS enzyme, or it can be recycled back to methionine using one of two enzymatic routes: MTHFR and MTR (5-methyltetrahydrofolate-homocysteine methyltransferase)/MTRR (5-Methyltetrahydrofolate-Homocysteine Methyltransferase Reductase), or BHMT (Betaine--Homocysteine S-Methyltransferase). Ideally homocysteine is balanced between being recycled back to methionine and going to transulfuration. Mutations on the CBS enzyme will cause homocysteine to be sucked down to transulfuration. Blood work will show low homocysteine, and taurine will be seen at high levels in urine. When there are mutations in MTHFR and MTR/MTRR or BHMT, homocysteine levels climb, as it is not being recycled back to methionine. See the "Genetic Test Analysis" section for more information on these mutations and how to support them.

Sulfoxidation Pathway

In this pathway, dietary sulfur is converted to sulfate. It detoxifies sulfites, which are used as a preservative. Those with a poorly functioning sulfoxidation system usually have an increased ratio of sulfite to sulfate in their urine. The strong odor in the urine after eating asparagus is due to poor sulfoxidation. The enzyme sulfite oxidase is dependent upon molybdenum and vitamin B1. A diet high in sulfites will deplete both of these.

Phase Three Detoxification

Phase three is the elimination phase where toxins from phase one and two leave the body. This happens through the kidneys to urine and through bile to stool. Some detoxification happens through the skin, also. When detoxification through bile and urine is not functioning optimally, we see more coming through the skin. This will manifest as skin conditions like acne, rashes, eczema, and others.

EGFR (Estimated glomerular filtration rate) will show whether the kidney's are functioning at optimal range. We want to see it above ninety. If it is below ninety, it is important to add in kidney support, like kidney flushes, herbs, glandulars, and juicing. I like Omega Alpha's Kidney Flush and Bell Kidney Cleanse Tea, and for juicing: apple, carrot, kale, parsley, fennel, cucumber, and a small number of beets and celery.

When bile flow is impaired, sunflower lecithin, taurine (if no active CBS mutation), bile salts, malic acid, mustard, chicory, and dandelion all promote bile flow. Liver flushes, castor oil packs, and coffee enemas also help greatly. One liver flush per month is ideal after support is put in place and continues until after gut work. At this point, doing three to four a year is good for maintenance. For coffee enemas, one to two a week is enough. Doing more than that can create dependency. I have seen a great many people become addicted to coffee enemas, and they feel terrible without them. If you have a sensitivity to caffeine or a CYP 1A2 mutation, then use a quarter dose of coffee. You can find instructions on how to do a liver flush in *The Amazing Liver and Gallbladder Flush* by Andreas Moritz, and coffee enema instructions are available online.

Once the body's nutrients are supported, it is important to add in binders. I usually wait until gut work, but if a person is presenting with diarrhea or loose stools in response to detoxification support, then adding them in sooner can help. I like to use zeolites, like Zeobind and Toxaprevent. Activated charcoal is only meant to be used occasionally, as it will pull nutrients. One to two times a week is plenty. I tend to stay away from fibers and pectin, unless SIBO has been ruled out.

Genetics Test Analysis

I have included this because I have had so many requests to do a summary of the genes I look at when doing genetics analyses. If it gets too scientific for you, skip over it. You can always come back to it another time or work with a practitioner to help you understand your genetics.

A basic understanding of genetics will help this make sense. -/- is no mutation, +/- is one mutation or heterozygous, and +/+ is two mutations or homozygous. Instead of mutation, I prefer to say this is someone's status. A person's status is not good or bad, but the word mutation makes it sound bad. Your status just shows which support you need and what you do not need.

We receive one set of genes from each parent. A mutation will cause either an upregulation or downregulation in the enzyme to which it corresponds. Enzymes cause reactions in the body. Upregulation speeds up the enzymes function. Downregulation slows down its function.

Not all mutations are active. Epigenetics states that gene mutations can turn on and off due to environmental factors. It is theorized that in good conditions and with proper tools, especially well-functioning methylation, the body has the ability to turn mutations on and off.

Genetics show us how a person will tend to react. Usually, when illness is present, there are active mutations present. Our genes have not changed much in the past hundred years, but the amount of stress and toxin exposure has greatly increased, which is the most likely cause of increased active mutations being seen. Below are the genes I look at. Let's start with understanding neurotransmitters.

The COMT enzyme breaks down the body's dopamine. A person with a COMT -/- status breaks down dopamine at a fast rate. A person who is COMT +/- breaks down dopamine at a medium rate, and COMT +/+ will break down dopamine at a slow rate. There really is no good or bad here. It is just knowing what you trend to so you can biohack and shift your brain chemistry using supplements. Dopamine is responsible for drive and motivation. Too much can cause OCD, aggression, and mania. Too little can cause depression, apathy, lack of focus, and lack of drive. We ideally want it to be in balance, but sometimes we may want to push to more dopamine to get things done, and at other times we may want to have less and be in a calm and more peaceful state.

When anxiety is present, I tend to have clients trend to a higher serotonin state. Serotonin is the happy, calming neurotransmitter. This is a better state for healing. Even when the person is COMT -/-, I will hold off building dopamine levels until proper mindset work is in place, to prevent the stress response from occurring and causing an increase in anxiety when dopamine levels are increased. Dopamine is broken down into adrenalin in times of stress. If a person is stuck in the anxiety/stress cycle, then building dopamine is contraindicated. Also, go-go-go is not a healing state. Even when someone is wanting extra energy, we want to shift to healing so the body can use the reserves we are rebuilding to heal instead of burning through them with daily tasks. Many people are addicted to high dopamine levels and being in the rat race. This requires mindset work and life changes. Turning inward is key.

COMT +/- individuals are often more balanced. They have decent drive and motivation and exhibit more peace. Other mutations can affect this, and we cannot look at one gene on its own. The key is looking at the full picture, which we will do below. These people will tolerate some methyl donors. Too much can lead to problems. We should see mid-range dopamine metabolites on an Organic Acids Test. If levels are high, it means the mutation is not active. If they are low, it indicates dopamine support is needed.

COMT +/+ individuals trend to high dopamine levels and are often overachievers and hyper focused. If their energy is not well channeled, it can lead to OCD, anxiety, and mania. Also, they are prone to sudden dopamine crashes and low serotonin levels. These individuals usually tolerate very few methyl donors. Adding in methyl donors will increase OCD and anxiety. I often see people come to me over-methylated, with anxiety through the roof due to over-methylating. It is so important to take a look at genetics and find out how much methyl donors are needed. COMT +/+ individuals should have low levels of dopamine metabolites on an Organic Acids Test. High levels indicate this mutation is not active.

COMT -/- individuals need a lot of methyl donors and dopamine support to keep up their drive and focus. Often, we see these individuals to be ADD. Focus just does not happen well without dopamine. Getting dopamine support on board when anxiety is under control is a game changer for them. Often ginkgo biloba is needed to slow dopamine breakdown. COMT -/- individuals should have high levels of dopamine metabolites on an Organic Acids Test. These people need a lot of methyl donors. If it is low, it indicates a need for dopamine support and methyl donors. Use caution when adding in methyl donors because even though a person has a need for them, if they have become very deficient for a long time, detoxification reactions will occur. COMT -/- people are prone to high levels of toxicity, as they tend to burn through their methyl donor and dopamine reserves.

The VDR (Vitamin D Receptor) Taq mutation affects vitamin D receptors. People with mutations here will need more vitamin D support and can benefit from rosemary and sage to assist with absorption. Having a mutation here will cause the person to be more sensitive to methyl donors and need less dopamine support. So, a COMT -/- individual with a VDR TAQ +/- can behave more like a COMT +/-. A COMT -/- individual with a VDR TAQ+/+ can behave more like COMT +/+. Chronically low vitamin D levels even in the presence of supplementation indicate the VDR TAQ is active.

MAOA (Monoamine oxidase) mutations slow the breakdown of serotonin. People who are MAO +/+ will break down serotonin slowly. Often if they are depressed, it is due to a lack of cofactors, like vitamin B6, magnesium, and zinc; it can also be due to other issues like low sex hormones, low dopamine, or existential crisis. We should see low levels of serotonin metabolites on an Organic Acids Test for people with this status. If they are high, it indicates it is not active. People who are MAO -/- will break down serotonin at a fast rate. We should see high levels on an Organic Acids Test. If levels are low, it indicates a lack of cofactors and precursors. These people need more serotonin support and are prone to depression, anxiety, and migraines. MAO +/- are often more balanced mood wise. They may need some serotonin support to prevent anxiety and depression.

MTHFR C677T. Everyone is obsessed with this one. On its own, it really does not give us that much information, except the person cannot convert folic acid to methylfolate (MTHF). It really is an easy fix. Supplement with MTHF. Even someone who is homozygous can still convert some folic acid to methylfolate. The enzyme is just not working as efficiently. The estimation is about twenty to forty percent less efficient for one active mutation and sixty-seventy percent for two mutations. The key to understanding genetics is to look at the full picture of all the listed mutations and see how they interact together. For example, someone who is COMT +/+ will tolerate few methyl donors. If they have a MTHFR C677T mutation, then care needs to be taken with how much MTHF they supplement. Too much will cause anxiety, OCD, migraines, etc. The detoxification pathways want the MTHF support, but the brain can only handle so much. Whenever starting any methyl donors, small doses are key, as is listening to and respecting the body's responses.

MTHFR A1298C mutation causes people to be more prone to higher ammonia levels. Ammonia requires two molecules of BH4 (Tetrahydrobiopterin) to be metabolized. Your brain requires BH4 to make neurotransmitters. This mutation plus an ammonia producing pathogen (or more than one) like Lyme, prevotella, or H. pylori can cause very high ammonia levels to build up in the body. Ammonia can cause brain fog, emotional issues due to neurotransmitter depletion from lack of BH4, vaginal issues, joint pain, and bladder issues. Couple it with an active CBS enzyme mutation, and lots of detoxification will be needed. What I see is people who run an Organic Acids Test often show low ammonia levels. Once we see these mutations and detoxification support is started, a rerun of Organic Acids Test will show very high ammonia. This was a game changer for my Interstitial Cystitis. One can use ornithine, molybdenum, BH4, royal jelly, and dandelion to help detoxify ammonia.

The BHMT enzyme is responsible for converting homocysteine back to methionine so it can be reused without going through MTHFR and MTR/MTRR enzymes. When MTHFR, MTR, and BHMT all have mutations, we tend to see very high homocysteine levels. A mutation on BHMT will slow its function. Two mutations slow it further and leads to high homocysteine levels. It is easily supported with phosphatidyl choline, ethanolamine, and serine. It is a great place to start supporting detoxification before adding in methyl donors, as it gets the methylation cycle rolling without causing too many problems.

A mutation on CBS C699T and 360T upregulate the CBS enzyme. It acts like a hole in the bucket. When you put methyl donors in, instead of going through methylation, it gets sucked down the drain. When the CBS enzyme is upregulated, we see high levels of sulfur and ammonia and high levels of taurine on an amino acid urine test. The problem is we do not see it until we put the methyl donors in. You do not know the bucket is leaking until you fill it with water. People with active CBS enzyme mutations are very sensitive to methyl donors and sulfur. This mutation, when active, needs to be addressed first. To check if it is active, run a homocysteine test. If it is below six, the odds are it is active. If it is above six, add in methyl donors and recheck in thirty days. A good indication it is active is a very bad reaction to the methyl donors. I use a reduced sulfur diet, dandelion tea, juicing, ornithine, molybdenum, and yarrow for four weeks, then add in methyl donors and retest homocysteine. Ideally, homocysteine should go up. If it does not, reduce methyl donors. An active CBS mutation can be difficult to get into balance.

MTR mutations upregulate activity of the MTR enzyme, which causes the person to burn through methyl B12 faster. These people are also prone to low lithium levels and support needs to be added in using lithium orotate. A common dose is 5 mg one to three times per day. Couple an MTR mutation with one or two MTRR mutations, and a person will have a great need for methyl B12. Mutations on MTRR cause the person to not be able to regenerate B12 efficiently. Always test vitamin B12 before supplementing. It is common for people with MTR mutations to have high levels of vitamin B12 even without supplementing because their lithium levels are low. Very commonly people using cyanocobalamin will have high levels of vitamin B12 as it is not being converted into usable vitamin B12. Caution needs to be used when adding in methyl B12 for people with COMT mutations and CBS mutations. When these mutations are present, hydroxocobalamin or adenosyl cobalamin are a better option with low dose methyl B12 used as tolerated.

CYP mutations affect phase one detoxification enzymes known as cytochrome p450. For the most part, they decrease the person's ability to detoxify drugs and toxins. What is really important to know is which herbs are contraindicated with certain mutations, as so many people take them on a daily basis. When phase one detoxification is slow, slowing it further is not ideal. Some key mutations follow. One or two mutations on CYP1A2 cause a person to be slow to metabolize caffeine. These people want to avoid curcumin and cumin in supplements and should not have grapefruit on a regular basis, as all these slow the enzyme further. One or two mutations on CYP3A4 slow the detoxification of drugs and hormones. These people should avoid quercetin, biopterin (black pepper), and milk thistle supplements. Grapefruit should also be avoided on a regular basis. All of these supplements will slow this enzyme further.

Organic Acids Test Analysis

The Organic Acids Test is the second of the foundation tests I run with all clients. It is best to read this section with your test in front of you so you can follow along. This analysis covers the Great Plains Organic Acids Test and will not convert to other tests. If you do not have your test results yet, skip over this section, and come back to it when you do. Page one of the results covers bacterial and fungal markers. Many practitioners run the test just to look at this page, and their client protocols are based on only this page. I do not. I have never found that approach to be successful and have seen hundreds of clients who have come to me from practitioners who took this approach with no success. It is normal in the beginning of the healing journey to have a bit of dysbiosis in bacteria and a mild overgrowth of yeast. Both of these are out of balance due to a weakened body. Throwing antifungals and antibacterial medications at someone in a weakened state, whether natural or not, will further weaken the body. It is counterproductive to healing. Remember, we are working to get the body stronger.

The only time I will do anything for bacteria or yeast is if I see many elevated markers. Then, I will get gentle support on board to tone down levels. I like Microbiome Labs Megamycobalance for yeast and Megaspore and Biocidin for bacteria.

Now scroll to page three of your results (as page two has some diagrams on mitochondria and neurotransmitters, which we will address later). On page three, the first thing we see is oxalates. See the "Oxalates" section in "Part One: Body" if your oxalate markers are high or you suspect oxalate issues.

Oxalates play a big role in many symptoms. Joint pain, IC, vaginal issues, and brain fog, to name a few. I choose Great Plains over other labs because their Organic Acids Test has this marker. When we see glycolic elevated, it indicates a predisposition to blood sugar issues. The thing with oxalates is often we do not catch them. The body goes through dumping phases and sometimes does not have the tools to detoxify, so often oxalates are not being released by the body at the time of the test. If a client is showing symptoms of high oxalates, and no oxalates are showing up, I will add in tools to detoxify and then retest.

Next are the glycolytic cycle metabolites. These are your first mitochondrial markers. Glycolysis is the first step of cellular respiration, which is how your body converts glucose from carbs and sugar in your diet to adenosine triphosphate, aka ATP. ATP is your body's fuel. When glycolysis is not functioning optimally due to lack of cofactors, dysfunction in mitochondria, or lack of oxygen, the body produces lactic acid and pyruvic acid. These are toxic substances in high amounts. Think if you have ever done a lot of exercise and got the burning in your muscles. That is lactic acid. Some people produce this at rest. This leads to fatigue, brain fog, and muscle weakness. For these people, carbs are not their ideal fuel until the mitochondria are repaired.

The Krebs cycle is the next step in cellular respiration. Here your body uses acetyl-CoA to form even more ATP. High markers here

238

indicate mitochondrial dysfunction. The amino acid metabolites from mitochondrial markers indicate problems converting amino acids from protein to energy.

Up next are the neurotransmitter markers. These markers only tell you what is going on if you have your genetics test results. These markers are the rate at which your body is breaking down your neurotransmitters, not the actual levels in the brain. For dopamine, we should see low levels for someone who is COMT +/+, fluctuating levels for COMT +/-, and high levels for someone who is COMT -/-. When someone is COMT +/+, we do not want to add dopamine precursors on a regular basis. There may be the odd occasion they need some support, but that is only if 5-HTP is not having the desired effect on depression. Low dopamine will present as apathy. For someone who is COMT -/-, if you see very low levels, it means they do not have enough cofactors or precursors. Cofactors are magnesium, P5P, and zinc. Precursors are DLPA, tyrosine, and macuna.

For serotonin metabolites, someone who is MAO -/- should have high levels of metabolites. We usually see low levels, as most people who are MAO -/- have burned through their cofactors and precursors due to high amounts of stress. A well supported brain with MAO -/- will show high levels. Cofactors are zinc, P5P, and magnesium. Precursors are tryptophan and 5-HTP. The problem with tryptophan is many people cannot convert it to 5-HTP, then to serotonin, due to dysfunction caused by pathogens and depleted cofactors. When someone cannot convert tryptophan to 5-HTP, we see high levels of quinolinic acid or a high quinolinic ratio to 5-HIAA on the Organic Acids Test. Supplementing with tryptophan is contraindicated in this case. St. John's Wort helps to slow breakdown of serotonin so that less 5-HTP is needed. St. John's Wort works as a natural SSRI (selective serotonin reuptake inhibitor), just without the side effects and withdrawal.

At the top of page four are folate markers. High markers here indicate issues with folate metabolism. Check MTHFR, BHMT, and MTR/MTRR mutations. I do not use this marker alone to determine supplements. Looking at blood work, the Organic Acids Test, and genetics alongside one another is key to getting a full picture.

Next up are ketone markers. We should only see these elevated in ketosis. When people have elevated markers here and are not intentionally putting themselves into ketosis, it shows problems with fat metabolism. Fat is not their ideal fuel until repair is complete.

The nutritional markers are up next and are self-explanatory. Low levels indicate the body needs more, and certain ones with a star can indicate the body needs more support when they are elevated. Vitamin C is almost always low on the Organic Acids Test from Great Plains. I do not recommend high dose ascorbic acid, as it can be converted to oxalates and cause a lot of issues. Ascorbic acid is added to foods as a preservative. It kills good and bad bacteria in high amounts. Ascorbic acid was one of the triggering factors of IC for me, as I was doing high dose vitamin C therapy. I prefer using whole food vitamin C support here, even if it is not sufficient to get this marker up.

On page five, we have our glutathione markers. For both NAC and glutathione, check for a CBS enzyme mutation before supplementing, as both are sulfur-based and can cause harm to those people who are sulfur sensitive. Hydrogen sulfide SIBO can also cause sulfur sensitivity, so use caution if you suspect it. A good indication is bloating and gas with a rotten egg smell when eating sulfur foods or high sulfur supplements.

The ammonia marker is very important, though like oxalates, it often shows low until support is in place because the body has run through its resources to detoxify. When we add support in and retest, we see it start to be eliminated. Ammonia causes a lot of symptoms like brain fog, IC, vaginal issues, joint pain, and extreme fatigue. I have found that people with Lyme, prevotella, and H. pylori have a higher ammonia burden, and detoxifying it provides a lot of relief to symptoms.

Marker 61 will appear elevated in people who are drinking aspartame. From this marker, I recently discovered that my client was drinking diet soda every night. It can also be due to an issue with salicylates or just high consumption of salicylates. If neither of those are the case, then GI bacteria is the cause.

The amino acid metabolites, when many are low, indicate poor protein absorption and/or poor protein breakdown. I add in protein powder and amino acid complexes to aid in elevating these markers.

Last is phosphoric acid. When low, it indicates low vitamin D. Correlate with blood work and VDR TAQ on genetics.

Blood Work Analysis

The next test I like to do is a full blood panel. CMP (Complete Metabolic Panel), CBC (Complete Blood Count), Lipid panel, iron panel, full thyroid panel, serum homocysteine, vitamin B12, and vitamin D3 give you a great picture of what is going on in your body. Again, it is best to have your labs in front of you for analysis when going through this section. If you do not have the results yet, skip over this section.

Many people go to their doctors, get blood work, and are told they are perfectly fine. It is frustrating for them because they feel something is wrong, or they do not feel their best. When doctors look at blood work, they are looking at disease ranges. The range is quite wide, and you only have something wrong when you get outside this range, according to the doctor. It is a sick care model. The ranges, themselves, are based on our unhealthy population. The ranges we want to look at are optimal ranges. This is where you want to be in order to feel your best. Remember my sister's blood work showing her ferritin was at 8 ug/L, and the doctors saying she was normal? She would feel much better with it between 70–90 ug/L. Optimal ranges are based on research in functional medicine looking at a healthy population. We want to look at our blood work and see what is outside of optimal range. This will show us what healing opportunities are available, by looking at what the possible causes are for those markers to be outside of optimal. Let's go over the markers and what they tell us. The ranges for the USA will be different from the rest of the world. I have included optimal ranges for the USA and International (IN), though some labs may use different units. Always check the units if you find your number is not correlating. The USA range will be listed first, followed by the International range. The reason USA is different is because it has not converted to metric. The blood work analysis comes from various courses and a book. Lisa Pomeroy's Functional Blood Analysis, Jim Marlowe's Understanding

Your Own Blood Test Results lecture, and *A Manual of Laboratory and Diagnostic Tests* by Frances Fischbach.

CMP (Complete Metabolic Panel)

Note in countries besides the USA, the below tests do not usually fall under "CMP." You will need to add them in separately. They may be called liver and kidney function tests. Sometimes, they do not have any label.

Marker	Possible Causes and Healing Opportunities	US Optimal Range	IN Optimal Range
Glucose	Levels that are too low show issues with low blood sugar or reactive hypoglycemia. Too high indicates vitamin B1 deficiency, liver congestion, metabolic syndrome, and as it gets higher, diabetes and insulin resistance. When levels are high, reducing processed carbs is a must. As levels increase, minimize grains. When glucose is above normal range, monitor insulin levels (optimal range 1–5 µIU/mL) and hemoglobin A1C (optimal range 4.5–5.5%) to rule out diabetes.	75–86 mg/dL	4.2–4.8 mmol/L
Phosphorus	High levels indicate bone growth or repair, too much vitamin D, poor kidney function, soda consumption, and decreased parathyroid function. Low indicates low stomach acid, high carb diets, alcohol use, diabetes, and overactive parathyroid.	3–4 mg/dL	0.97–1.30 mmol/L
EGFR	When below 90, it indicates decreased kidney function. Support with juicing and Bell Kidney Cleanse Tea. It does not indicate kidney disease unless other markers in the CMP that show decreased kidney function correlate.	>90	>90

Uric Acid	High levels indicate gout, kidney issues, oxidative stress, mold, and inflammation. Tart cherry extract and non-aluminum baking soda help lower levels. For acidity on any of the below markers, use baking soda at a dose of 1/8–1/4 tsp in a glass of water on an empty stomach, 1–3x per day or 1–5x per week. Low levels indicate poor detoxification, low molybdenum, low folate, and B12 deficiency. Explore those issues.	3–6 mg/dL	178–350 umol/L
BUN (Blood Urea Nitrogen)	Low levels indicate poor liver and pancreatic function and poor protein absorption and utilization. For liver dysfunction, see "Detoxification Pathways" section. Adding in pancreatic enzymes at the end of meals, working on detoxification, and increasing protein intake through protein powders, amino acids, meat, and raw milk will help bring this to optimal range. High levels indicate kidney dysfunction, low stomach acid, dehydration, dysbiosis, and too much protein. Correlate with further testing to determine appropriate action.	12–17 mg/dL	12–17 mg/dL
Creatinine	Low levels indicate poor protein absorption and utilization and lack of exercise. Use same action as that of low BUN. High indicates renal dysfunction (correlate with other kidney markers), too much protein, and dehydration. Dehydration is common after fasting and is the usual cause when high.	8–1.1 mg/dL	70.7–97.2 umol/L
Sodium	High levels indicate Cushing's disease, dehydration, and high cortisol. Low indicates low cortisol, Addison's disease, and fluid loss. Run a DUTCH Test check cortisol levels.	135–142 mmol/L	135–142 mmol/L

Potassium	High levels indicate acidity, low cortisol, and dehydration. Low indicates high cortisol, too alkaline, high blood pressure, and high cortisol.	4–4.5 mmol/L	4–4.5 mmol/L
Chloride	High levels indicate acidity, high cortisol, and dehydration. Low indicates low cortisol, alkaline, (for alkalinity increase fruits or use lemon in water daily or 1–3x per week), low stomach acid, and fluid loss.	100–106 mmol/L	100–106 mmol/L
CO2	High levels indicate too alkaline, high cortisol, and low stomach acid. Low indicates vitamin B1 deficiency (use benfotiamine, fat-soluble vitamin B1 as it is very usable by the body, 300–600 mg per day), too acidic, and low cortisol. Run a DUTCH Test.	25–28 mmol/L	25–28 mmol/L
Calcium	High levels indicate too much vitamin D supplementation, as vitamin D aids in calcium absorption, low thyroid, and hyper parathyroid (if you suspect parathyroid issues see your doctor). Low indicates low magnesium, calcium, vitamins K and D, and low stomach acid. Raw milk with vitamins D and K in the morning is great for increasing calcium levels.	9.5–10 mg/dL	2.37–2.50 mmol/L
Protein	High levels indicate dehydration and liver dysfunction. Low indicates poor protein absorption and utilization, low stomach acid, and liver dysfunction.	6.9–7.4 g/dL	69–74 g/L
Albumin	High levels indicate dehydration and liver dysfunction. Low indicates oxidative stress, liver dysfunction, low stomach acid, and vitamin C deficiency. For vitamin C deficiency, use camu camu berry or another natural vitamin C, as ascorbic acid can increase oxalates.	4–5 g/dL	40–50 g/L

Globulin	High levels indicate liver dysfunction, heavy metal burden (see "Heavy Metal Detoxification" section in "Part One: Body"), low stomach acid, and oxidative stress. Juicing apple, carrot, kale, and other low oxalate veggies helps. If you do not have any issues with sulfur, adding in sulforaphane can help. Low indicates inflammation and immune insufficiency. When I see immune deficiency, I add in spleen and thymus glandulars.	2.4–2.8 g/dL	24–28 g/L
Bilirubin	High levels indicate poor bile flow and liver dysfunction, Gilbert's Syndrome, oxidative stress, and thymus dysfunction (add in thymus glandular). Low indicates that spleen support is needed (add in spleen glandular).	0.2–1 mg/dL	3.42–17.10 umol/L
Alkaline phosphatase	High levels indicate liver and bile dysfunction, bone changes, and estrogen or contraceptive use. Low indicates low zinc.	70–100 IU/L	70–100 IU/L
LDH (Lactate dehydrogenase)	High levels indicate liver and bile dysfunction, B12 and folate deficiency, cardiovascular disease, high viral load, and inflammation. Low indicates low blood sugar, oxalates, and poor carbohydrate metabolism.	140–200 IU/L	140–200 IU/L
AST (aspartate aminotransferase) and ALT (alanine aminotransferase)	High levels indicate liver and cardiovascular dysfunction, medication use, gut inflammation, viral infections, vitamin E deficiency, and alcoholism. Low indicates B6 deficiency. When liver enzymes are elevated, I use a product called Flor-Essence Gentle Detox For The Whole Body. It is safe for all genetics. If a person does not have any CYP mutations, it is okay to do a basic liver support. Most basic liver supports contain milk thistle and turmeric, which are contraindicated for some people. See "Genetics Test Analysis" section.	10–25 IU/L	10–25 IU/L

GGT (gamma-glutamyl transferase)	High levels indicate liver and pancreatic dysfunction, alcoholism, excess iron, viral infections, and medication use. High levels of GGT depletes glutathione. If high, support with liposomal, topical, or reduced glutathione. Glutathione is a sulfur amino acid, so use caution if sulfur issues are present. Low can be caused by birth control pills, vitamin B6 deficiency, and magnesium deficiency.	18–28 IU/L	18–28 IU/L

*Remember that many people cannot convert vitamin B6 from food to the active form P5P due to poor gut flora and conversion issues. Supplementing with P5P is ideal if high B6 levels are found when supplementing with B6. P5P will flush out the unconverted B6. Use caution when starting P5P. Low doses are best, as some people do not tolerate it well, especially people with prior or current use of benzodiazepines. People with pyroluria will often have a detoxification reaction to P5P. A quarter of a 25 mg capsule, or just a sprinkle, is the best place to start; then, slowly increase. A good top dose is 25 mg, as the body can only absorb so much at a time due to first pass metabolism. It will end up in the urine.

CBC (Complete Blood Count)

Marker	Possible Causes and Healing Opportunities	US Optimal Range	IN Optimal Range
White Blood Cells (WBC)	High levels indicate acute infection or stress. Low indicates chronic infection, pancreatic insufficiency, autoimmune disorders, reduced bone marrow production, and raw food diets. When levels are low, use myrrh to support WBC production and supplement or eat bone marrow. Use pancreatic enzymes at the end of meals to support digestion and prevent WBC from having to break up undigested food. For high levels, support the immune system with echinacea and elderberry.	5–7.5 x10^3/µL	5–7.5 x10^9/L
Red Blood Cells	High levels indicate dehydration and respiratory disorders. Low indicates deficiencies in: iron, B12, folate, *copper, and vitamin C. Low also indicates internal bleeding. Use genetics to determine ideal B12 and confirm on blood work that B12 is low. Check homocysteine and genetics to see if there is need for folate supplementation.	3.9–4.9 x10^6/µL	3.9–4.9 x10^9/L
Hemoglobin	High levels indicate dehydration and respiratory disorders. Low indicates deficiencies in: iron, B12, folate, copper, and vitamin C. Low also indicates internal bleeding (often due to ulcers or heavy periods in women). Rule out ulcers and heavy periods with doctor if levels are very low. In pregnancy, hemoglobin will be lower, as blood volume increases to accommodate the fetus.	13.5–15 g/dL	135–150 g/L

Hematocrit	High levels indicate dehydration and respiratory disorders. Low indicates deficiencies in: iron, B12, folate, copper, and vitamin C. Low can also indicate internal bleeding and thymus dysfunction. Supplement with desiccated thymus and any nutrients found to be deficient.	37–48%	37–48%
Mean Corpuscular Volume (MCV)	High levels indicate deficiencies in: B12, folate, and vitamin C. Low indicates iron and B6 deficiencies. Low can also indicate internal bleeding.	82–89.9 fL	82–89.9 fL
Mean Corpuscular Hemoglobin (MCH)	High levels indicate B12 and folate deficiencies, as well as low stomach acid. Rule out H. pylori before supplementing with HCL, as increasing stomach acid causes the bacteria to burrow deeper into the stomach lining, making it harder to eradicate. Low indicates internal bleeding, deficiencies in: vitamin B6, vitamin C, and iron. Low can also indicate heavy metal toxicity.	28–31.9 pg	28–31.9 pg
Mean Corpuscular Hemoglobin Concentration (MCHC)	High levels indicate B12 and folate deficiencies, as well as low stomach acid. Low indicates deficiencies in: iron, vitamin B6, and vitamin C. Low also indicates a high heavy metal burden.	32–35 g/dL	320–350 g/L
Red Cell Distribution Width (RDW)	High levels indicate deficiencies in: iron, B12, and folate. High levels also indicate anemia. Low indicates acute or chronic infection, as well as inflammation.	11–13%	11–13%
Platelets	High levels indicate atherosclerosis. Low indicates heavy metals and oxidative stress. Too high or too low can indicate some forms of cancer. Some people genetically have lower or higher levels. Rule out cancer with a doctor.	150–385 x10³/μL	150–385 x10⁹/ μL
Neutrophils	High levels indicate chronic or acute infection, as well as inflammation. Low indicates chronic infection and blood disorders.	40–60%	40–60%

Lymphocytes	High levels indicate chronic or acute infection, inflammation, and toxin overload. Low indicates oxidative stress, chronic or acute infection, cancer, autoimmune issues, medications, low bone marrow production, and deficiencies in zinc and protein.	24–44%	24–44%
Monocytes	High levels indicate liver dysfunction, parasites, recovery from infection, and inflammation. Low indicates poor bone marrow production, autoimmune conditions, medications use, and deficiencies in B12 and folate.	0–7%	0–7%.
Eosinophils	High levels indicate parasites and inflammation.	0–3%	0–3%
Basophils	High levels indicate inflammation, parasites, and high histamine.	0–1%	0–1%

*When it comes to copper, it is best to run a Great Plains Copper Zinc Test before supplementing, as many people are copper toxic and deficient at the same time. When ceruloplasmin is too low to transport the copper to the cells, supplementing with animal source vitamin A (like cod liver) helps to increase it. Too much zinc and vitamin D, as well as citrate forms of supplements, can also lower ceruloplasmin. More is not better. The Great Plains Copper Zinc Test is the test I prefer, as it shows non-ceruloplasmin copper.

Lipid Panel

Marker	Possible Causes and Healing Opportunities	US Optimal Range	IN Optimal Range
Cholesterol	High levels indicate chronic infection, inflammation, low thyroid, liver and cardiovascular dysfunction, poor bile flow, and poor metabolism of fats. Low indicates oxidative stress, poor bile flow and absorption of fats, liver dysfunction, manganese deficiency, heavy metals, and autoimmune conditions. For low levels, increase good fats from olive oil, avocado, clean meats, eggs, butter, ghee, and raw milk. For high cholesterol, use plant sterols and red rice yeast. Sunflower lecithin and bile salts help with fat breakdown and absorption. Taurine for people who have low levels will help with bile flow. When using taurine, rule out CBS issues, and be cautious if you have issues with sulfur. See phase three detoxification in the "Detoxification Pathways" section to help with bile flow.	170–200 mg/dL	4.4–5.2 mmol/L
Triglycerides	High levels indicate blood sugar dysregulation, liver and cardiovascular dysfunction, poor bile flow, H. pylori, birth control use, alcohol use, and hypothyroidism. Low indicates liver dysfunction, poor bile flow, and autoimmune conditions.	70–80 mg /dL	0.79–0.90 mmol/L
HDL Cholesterol (high-density lipoprotein)	High levels indicate possible autoimmune conditions. Low indicates poor bile flow, liver dysfunction, lack of exercise, H. pylori, hypothyroidism, heavy metals, and oxidative stress.	55–85 mg/dL	1.4–2.2 mmol/L
LDL Cholesterol (low-density lipoprotein)	High levels indicate poor bile flow, liver dysfunction, lack of exercise, H. pylori, hypothyroidism, heavy metals, and oxidative stress. Low indicates oxidative stress, chronic infection, and inflammation.	80–100 mg/dL	2.1–2.6 mmol/L

Iron Panel

This should be fasting blood work, with a ten to twelve hour fast. You should be off iron supplements for ten days.

Marker	Possible Causes and Healing Opportunities	US Optimal Range	IN Optimal Range
Iron serum	High levels indicate iron overload and or hemochromatosis. It can also indicate conversion problems if ferritin is low and iron serum is high. When this is the case, focus on phase two detoxification pathways. It can also be high when consuming a lot of red meats or cooking with cast iron pans. Low levels indicate iron deficiency anemia. This can be caused by low stomach acid. In women, it can be due to heavy periods. Whole food vitamin C helps absorption.	85–130 ug/dL	15–23 umol/L
Total Iron Binding Capacity (TIBC)	The best way to explain this test is that iron needs to be transported by red blood cells. Iron binds to oxygen. Transferrin is the taxi, and TIBC is a measure of transferrin. It is showing how much your body can transport. If it is high, it indicates iron deficiency or bleeding. When it is low, it indicates overload.	250–350 ug/dL	45–63 umol/L
Percent saturation	This indicates how many spots in the taxi are filled. When high, it indicates iron overload. Liver disease, alcoholism, and cancer can also cause this to be high. Low indicates iron deficiency.	25–30%	25–30%

Ferritin	Ferritin is your body's iron stores. High levels indicate iron overload. If this is above optimal range, it is good to give blood and rule out hemochromatosis. Inflammation can elevate ferritin, even with normal serum levels. There is a theory that the body will store iron to keep it away from pathogens. Low ferritin indicates iron deficiency and possible iron deficiency anemia if hemoglobin is low. If ferritin is below nine, iron sucrose shots may be needed to elevate it. I do not believe in avoiding supplementing with iron so as not to feed pathogens. So many symptoms like dizziness, weakness, and fatigue can be caused by low iron. I have found the best way to increase iron is with grass fed beef liver and iron bisglycinate supplements. Some people are sensitive to glycine, especially those on benzodiazepines. If this is the case, eating small amounts of grass fed, well sourced beef liver is the best option. Eat small amounts each day with natural vitamin C. Grass fed beef liver also has a whole complement of cofactors and nutrients. It is one of our super foods, and it is a shame that society rarely eats it now. Remember that the liver in the grocery store or at restaurants are different. Conventional cows have high toxin burdens, much of which will have passed through their livers. There is actually a totally different odor from conventional liver to grass fed, well sourced liver. The odor of conventional liver can clear a house. Grass fed liver barely has an odor.	70–90 ng/mL	90–110 ug/L

Thyroid Panel

Marker	Possible Causes and Healing Opportunities	US Optimal Range	IN Optimal Range
TSH (thyroid-stimulating hormone)	This range is quite a bit smaller than the normal range. This is a feel-good range. If you are on Natural Desiccated Thyroid (NDT), TSH should be lower, as the brain is sensing the thyroid hormone and turning off production. High TSH is indicative of primary hypothyroidism. The brain is sensing there is not enough thyroid hormone, so is saying, "Thyroid, produce more please." When TSH is low, it indicates hyperthyroid. This can also be due to pituitary and hypothalamus issues.	0.5–2 µIU/mL	IN 0.5–2 MU/L
Free and Total T4	High levels indicate hyperthyroidism. Medications can cause this to be elevated. Low indicates hypothyroidism and iodine deficiency.	Total T4 6.0–11.9 µg/dL Free T4 1.4–1.8 ng/dL	Total T4 77–153 nmol/L Free T4 18–23 pmol/L
Total and Free T3	High levels indicate hyperthyroidism or pooling due to low iron and cortisol dysfunction. Iodine deficiency can also cause high T3. Low indicates selenium deficiency and hypothyroidism.	Total T3 120–180 ng/dL Free T3 3.4–4.4 pg/mL	Total T3 120–180 ng/dL Free T3 5.2–6.8 pmol/L

Reverse T3 (rT3)	When elevated, it means the body is wanting to rest and heal. It indicates issues with inflammation, stress, and chronic infections. Trauma and emotional stress can elevate it. Iron and selenium deficiencies and certain medication can also cause it to be elevated. When above fifteen, NDT will often make people feel worse. Most NDT given will be converted to rT3. To lower rT3, a doctor may prescribe free T3 only. In my opinion, it is best to first rebuild the body, rebalance systems, repair detoxification, and remove stress. If it is still high after doing gut work, then consider flushing with T3. I believe the body has a reason for doing things. If it wants to rest, adding in more T3 to give energy to daily tasks is against its wishes. Support and listen to the body.	<15	<15
Thyroid Antibodies	High levels indicate an autoimmune response. I start with Moducare. The phytosterols are known for their immune modulating capabilities. They do take three to six plus months to work. If rT3 is below fifteen, NDT can be started, as that will often turn off the autoimmune response. Working on detoxification pathways and removing internal stress are the most important steps to turning off the immune response.	Thyroglobulin <20 Thyroid Peroxidase <10	Thyroglobulin <20 Thyroid Peroxidase <10

Additional Markers

Marker	Possible Causes and Healing Opportunities	US Optimal Range	IN Optimal Range
Serum homocysteine	I like serum testing for homocysteine, as I have found plasma to not always correlate. This is a very important marker. When low, it often indicates a CBS enzyme mutation is active. When high, it indicates that homocysteine is not being recycled into methionine. From genetics, we know that this can be due to more than just MTHFR. Knowing your genetics is important. BHMT, MTR/ MTRR, and MTHFR C677T can all cause homocysteine to be high. Often, people see a high homocysteine and assume it means MTHFR, so they supplement with MTHF. This can cause more issues for people who are COMT +/+, and often it is not even MTHFR causing the issue. It is currently such a big topic that everyone assumes they have it and are supplementing with high doses of MTHF and over methylating. I have found that many people do not have any mutation, and those that do, the mutation is only heterozygous. Remember, a mutation does not mean the enzyme is not functioning, just that it is either functioning too fast or too slow, depending on which mutation we are discussing. If homocysteine is low, make sure to check CBS mutations, and be cautious adding in methyl donors.	6–7.2 umol/L	6–7.2 umol/L

Vitamin D	Vitamin D is used to help the body absorb calcium from the diet (along with vitamin K, which helps it get into our bones). The best source of vitamin D is from the sun. Wearing sunscreen will prevent absorption. Practice sun safety, instead, by keeping exposure time to less than burn time. Seek shade and cover up with loose, white clothing, if needed. Whatever chemicals you put on your skin will end up in your body. I am not a fan of high dose vitamin D therapy, except for certain conditions like MS. Slowly working up to 5000 IU vitamin D with 200 mcg total vitamin K is how I do it. Some people do not tolerate that dose. Always listen to your body on the ideal dose. Check VDR TAQ, as mutations here can make a person burn through vitamin D faster. Rosemary and sage help with absorption and utilization. I take vitamins D and K with my glass of raw milk in the morning.	60–80 ng/mL	150–200 nmol/L
Vitamin B12	When testing B12, make sure to be off it for 7–10 days to ensure we are seeing what you are retaining. You can also test while taking it, to make sure you are absorbing it. Knowing your COMT status and VDR TAQ will determine which form to take. COMT mutations and VDR TAQ mutations will increase sensitivity to methyl donors. If you have these mutations and MTR or MTRR mutations, supplement mostly with hydroxy or adenosyl B12, and add in very small doses of methyl B12 at a low frequency. I will often use drops of sublingual B12, so clients are able to titrate up from 100 mcg to 1000 mcg. If it is causing a reaction, only use a few times a week. As the brain is balanced with amino acid therapy, you can often increase methyl donors. Remember that active CBS mutations may make a person very sensitive to methyl donors, too. If CBS is active, methyl donors are contraindicated, as they will just cause elevated ammonia and sulfur levels as they are shunted down transsulfuration.	800–900 pg/mL	590–664 pmol/L

DUTCH Test Analysis

On the DUTCH (Dried Urine Test for Comprehensive Hormones) Test adrenal and sex hormone portions, I like to look at the diagrams. They look like little clocks. Optimal range is between ten and two on the clock.

The reason the DUTCH Test is best to check adrenals is that it shows free cortisol, a cortisol curve, and metabolized cortisol. Metabolized cortisol is important. Many people run a saliva test, believe they have low cortisol based on the results from saliva testing, and begin taking things to boost cortisol, like glandulars and adrenal cortex. Many times, these people would have seen high metabolized cortisol on the DUTCH Test. The problem is not adrenal output. The problem is the body is inactivating free cortisol to cortisone, which is the body's anti-inflammatory; or it is breaking free cortisol down quickly. By taking glandulars or cortex, they are turning off adrenal function and creating a dependency on the glandular or medication. I rarely see true adrenal fatigue, where both free and metabolized cortisol are low. When that pattern presents, it is usually along with low DHEA and other hormones. Boosting those levels with hormone support with pregnenolone, DHEA, and progesterone is a better first line of action.

Adrenal support in the form of herbs is great, too. The most common presentation with fatigue is low free cortisol and high metabolized cortisol. This indicates stress on the body, as well as inflammation. Licorice can be used to slow breakdown of cortisol, but caution is needed with high blood pressure. It is also important to listen to the body's wisdom. It is inactivating cortisol for a reason. It wants rest. Going against its wishes is counterproductive. It is best to only use as needed and honor the body. Work to remove the stress on the body.

Another pattern is high free cortisol to low metabolized cortisol. People with this pattern often present with high anxiety levels. Because metabolized cortisol is low, it is contraindicated to lower free cortisol with herbs. Mindset, neurotransmitter support, meditation, and lifestyle changes are used to bring down cortisol with this pattern.

Another common pattern is high free and metabolized cortisol. When this pattern is present and the anxiety/stress response is being felt, the supplements Seriphos or Enerphos can be used to lower levels. Anytime support is added in for adrenals or sex hormones, it is important to retest in sixty to ninety days to monitor how the support is working for the body and whether it is still needed.

Another common pattern is good free and good metabolized cortisol. It is quite comical how often a person presents with fatigue as a symptom, and their adrenals look great. It shows the importance of testing. Fatigue does not automatically mean adrenals are not working. Often it is not the adrenals at all. If it is, then it is adrenal dysfunction. The last thing to look at when looking at the adrenals is the cortisol curve.

This curve shows circadian rhythm. The optimal curve will be in the middle of the high and low ranges. There should be more cortisol in the morning, lower in the afternoon, and then lowest at night. It is higher in the morning to give energy to start the day and slowly decreases toward bedtime so a person can sleep. Any spike or drop where it is not meant to be can create symptoms. A spike in nighttime free cortisol is usually due to using technology at night and a poor circadian rhythm. Turning off blue light emitting technology and using relaxation techniques is key to addressing it, along with waking up earlier in the mornings.

A spike during the day will be in response to a stressor. This often presents as anxiety, heart racing, and an inability to calm down. A spike in morning cortisol is due to pathogens and detoxification during the night. We do not want to turn off this response. We want to move to gut work and address the pathogens. It is common to see extremely low levels in the morning when a person is going to bed late and waking late. Slowly moving wake up times to earlier is key to addressing this pattern, though it can take months of getting up earlier for the body to want to go to bed earlier. The free and metabolized cortisol patterns need to be considered when choosing to support the adrenals with supplements or herbs or to use lifestyle modification to help.

The hormone portion interpretation will be different for cycling females, post-menopausal females, and males.

For cycling females, the test is taken days nineteen-twenty-one of a twenty-eight to thirty-day cycle. For women with irregular cycles, an ovulation kit is needed to determine the LH (luteinizing hormone) surge. When the surge happens, continue testing to see when the surge decreases. You can run the DUTCH Test five to seven days after the decrease occurs on the LH test. The LH surge indicates ovulation is coming; it does not indicate ovulation has occurred. I remember when I was testing to get pregnant. I had my LH surge on Saturday; by Thursday there was still no ovulation, and LH was still high. Cervical fluid can also be monitored. Peak ovulation, egg white fluid indicates the day before ovulation. The day after ovulation, fluid will begin to decrease. Some women can have fertile egg white cervical fluid for five to seven days prior to ovulating, though those with high levels of fertile fluids usually have a more regular cycle.

At the top of the DUTCH Test, you will see estrogen, progesterone, and testosterone levels listed. In the adrenal portion, note the DHEA. These are the total levels. It is good to note this information, and then proceed to the third page. Estrogen and progesterone levels change throughout the month, depending on the phase of the cycle. Estrogen rises to stimulate ovulation and then slowly decreases, whereas progesterone rises after ovulation because it is used to grow and maintain the uterine lining to support a possible pregnancy. If fertilization of the egg does not occur, both levels fall, which stimulates menstruation. When testing in the luteal phase before a period, progesterone levels should be higher than estrogen levels.

If estrogen is higher than progesterone levels, it signifies estrogen dominance. When this happens, especially when metabolism on page three is not optimal, it needs to be addressed first. Any bioidentical hormone support can cause further estrogen dominance. DIM (Dindolylmethane) and CDG (Calcium D-Glucarate) are great for bringing estrogen into balance. Use DIM with caution if you have sulfur issues. If sulfur is an issue, it is best to address that first.

On page three of the DUTCH Test, there is a pie chart showing estrogen metabolism. It shows how well your body is detoxifying estrogen. The green is 2-OH, which is safely detoxified. The blue is 16-OH, which is neutral. The red is 4-OH, which is unsafe metabolites. When red levels are high, the body is not metabolizing estrogen well. DIM helps bring this into range by working on the pathways in the liver that are used to metabolize estrogen. It speeds up detoxification and helps send the estrogen down the 2-OH pathway. When 16-OH is high, it indicates gut dysbiosis. CDG helps, as does gut work. Ideally, the ratios should be eighty percent green, ten percent blue, and ten percent red.

At the bottom of the third page, estrogen methylation is shown. This is a great indicator of how well your genetics and phase two support are working. For progesterone levels, it is best to see the little clock on page one around two o'clock for optimal. If they are low, support first with chaste tree berry (vitex). Since all the support is on board from the foundation tests, the body should have the resources to make progesterone. This is a safe option when estrogen dominance or issues with detoxification of estrogen are present. Chaste tree tells the brain to increase production of progesterone. Some women do well taking it from the time of ovulation until their period; other women use it all month. If chaste tree does not help increase levels on a retest, and there is no estrogen dominance, or if estrogen dominance is supported with herbs, then bioidentical progesterone can be used up to 200 mg per day from two days after ovulation until the start of menstruation. Higher doses can delay menstruation and feed estrogen levels. Many symptoms can occur at higher doses. Progesterone can be used orally, vaginally, or on the skin. If low beta progesterone levels are present, taking it orally before bed can help with sleep. Most women prefer to use it vaginally. There are many lower dosage over the counter topicals available. Personally, I like Biomatrix Nutrition's progesterone, as it comes in a dropper and can be used orally or topically, and it is easily titrated. It has natural ingredients. The downside to these over-the-counter ones is that for women needing the 200 mg, they will be going through a lot. Often, though, it is less work than trying to get a prescription. For retesting hormone levels, see DUTCH Test educational videos on their website.

When chronic fatigue is present, often low DHEA and low hormones overall will be evident. If no estrogen dominance or poor metabolism is present, DHEA and pregnenolone can be used to raise levels. I prefer this as a last line of defense. It is better to turn on the body's ability to make its own rather than give it the hormones. In some cases, it is needed due to extremely low levels of hormones and a person not responding to herbs and supplements. This support is then used to help the body through gut work. Douglas Labs has great sublingual DHEA and pregnenolone. When using hormone supplements, retesting using the DUTCH Test needs to be done every three months to check detoxification pathways. Start with up to 25 mg of pregnenolone, and if needed, add in 25 mg of DHEA. Always start low, and only use what is needed. If you have any side effects, decrease to a dose that is tolerated.

Testosterone levels and metabolites are also important. Common with PCOS (Polycystic ovary syndrome) is high testosterone or high androgen metabolites. Douglas Labs TestoQuench (TQ) for women is a great product to use when free or metabolized levels are high. Often, people want to raise testosterone levels because free levels are showing low. It is important to see the metabolites for this reason, as alpha androsterone levels are much more potent than testosterone. High androgen levels present as acne, greasy hair, male pattern hair loss, deepening of the voice, decreased breast size, and facial hair in women. Herbs like saw palmetto, nettle, pygeum, and pumpkin seed all help lower levels and support healthy metabolism of androgens. Prostate formulas for men, when taken in lower doses, can help women presenting with high androgens. For low testosterone in women, regulating estrogen and progesterone levels, plus supporting the body, are the best options.

Men can take the test at any time. For sex hormones, we are looking for any signs of estrogen dominance or poor breakdown of estrogen. When either are present, DIM and CDG are helpful. The range of testosterone for men by age can be found on the test. I have found men feel best with their testosterone at two to three on the little clock.

Before boosting testosterone levels, it is important to check metabolism. High metabolites, especially high alpha DHT levels, make raising free levels contraindicated. Alpha DHT is very potent and when high, testosterone lowering is needed, as it can lead to prostate inflammation, aggression, anger, and male cancers. It is quite common for men to be prescribed testosterone based on free levels for symptoms of low drive, depression, and low energy. Often these men have issues with metabolism and have high DHT. This can lead to a lot of damage. Always test with a DUTCH Test before using bioidenticals. Often symptoms are due to low neurotransmitter levels or an existential crisis such as lack of purpose, not low testosterone. Herbs like saw palmetto, nettle, pygeum, pumpkin seed, and lycopene all help with high metabolites and also bring down alpha DHT levels. If both free testosterone and metabolites are low, herbs like horny goat weed and Tribulus can be used successfully to raise levels. Using herbs to raise low testosterone would be my first line of action before using testosterone, itself. If DHEA levels, free testosterone, and metabolites are all low and herbal support does not help on a retest, then using pregnenolone and DHEA can help. First use pregnenolone; then, use DHEA, if needed, up to 25 mg. Retest every three months to monitor metabolism. If there are no improvements, adding in testosterone bioidenticals would be my next step.

For post-menopausal women or women who have had a hysterectomy, testing can be done at any time. It is still important to check hormone levels, especially metabolism, if bioidentical hormones will be used for support. Progesterone and estrogen should be in the purple band called post-menopausal range. Often testosterone, testosterone metabolites, and DHEA are still high. This is common with women who have had PCOS. If support is needed for high levels, see the high testosterone and metabolite option for women above. Lower doses taken less frequently can be used. Many women who are post-menopausal feel better on bioidentical support. The goal is not to bring levels to a cycling woman's range but to just support the body. It is especially important to check 4-OH levels and estrogen methylation. When estrogen levels are in the post-menopausal range, high 4-OH is nominal because overall levels are so low. If a person has high 4-OH and adds in bioidentical estradiol, they can run into problems with toxic estrogen. DIM and CGD can be taken if estradiol bioidenticals are used and 4-OH is trending high. DIM and CDG are contraindicated with exceptionally low total estrogen levels, as they will lower estrogen further. If progesterone support is used, it is important to monitor estrogen and estrogen metabolites, as progesterone can be converted to estrogen. Estriol is a safe form of estrogen that has already been broken down. It can be used vaginally to help with dryness for women who are post-menopausal. It is often not enough to help with hot flashes. Vaginal DHEA is a great option for vaginal dryness. For women who have had a hysterectomy, bioidenticals can be used in higher levels to bring them up to the cycling woman's range until the age where menopause would have occurred, at which time doses can be lowered. Monitor hormones every six months to a year. Estradiol is only available via prescription, and it is best to work with a Naturopathic Doctor or Functional Medicine Doctor to monitor levels when using it or higher doses of progesterone.

The last page of the test shows organic acids markers. The interpretation is the same as the corresponding markers from the Organic Acids Test. Markers for melatonin and oxidative stress are also found on the last page. For melatonin, I do not like to use high doses when levels are low. Even a small dose of 0.25 mg will show as a huge increase on the DUTCH Test. Taking high doses can cause drowsiness the following morning. One milligram before bed to help with falling asleep or a 1 mg timed release to help stay asleep is more than enough. For high oxidative stress, juicing is a great option. Sulforaphane is great when there are no sulfur or ammonia issues. The remaining Organic Acids Test markers are addressed the same as in the "Organic Acids Test Analysis" section.

ACKNOWLEDGMENTS

This book would not have been possible without the support of my amazing husband Eric. We make a great team. I am so grateful to be spending my life with you.

Special thanks to Keidi Keating, Miranda Baka, Tabatha Farnel, and Michelle Burbidge for helping me with editing.

Photo Credit: Thank you to Meg Davey for the beautiful picture of Kaiden and I.